Lupus And Me: Living Well With An Autoimmune Illness:
Healthy Nutrition

Jenn Schoch, RN, BA, MSN, FNP-BC

Family Nurse Pra

D1553416

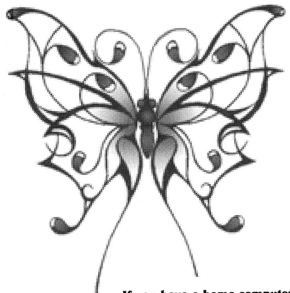

Note to Readers:

Legal Disclaimer

The information in this book represents the author's opinions, and is not intended to replace medical advice. This book is not intended to provide medical advice, or to be a substitute for medical advice from your personal physician. Before beginning this, or any other nutritional program, consult your physician first, to be sure it is appropriate for you.

The author has made every effort to supply accurate information in the creation of this book. The information in this book is not intended to diagnose, prescribe, treat, cure, or prevent any disease. Neither this, nor any other book should be used as a substitute for professional medical advice or treatment.

Neither the author, nor the publisher, shall be liable for any loss, injury, or damage caused, or alleged to be caused, directly or indirectly from any information or suggestion in this book. The statements in this book have not been evaluated by the U.S. Food and Drug Administration.

Dedication

To my soulmate and partner, Emily, who understands that the journey is long, but worth the ride! Thank you! I could never have done this without your encouragement, patience, and support. See Emily's recipes for Bone Broth in Chapter 4.

I also would like to thank Tambra, for all of your help and support—you have been a huge help!

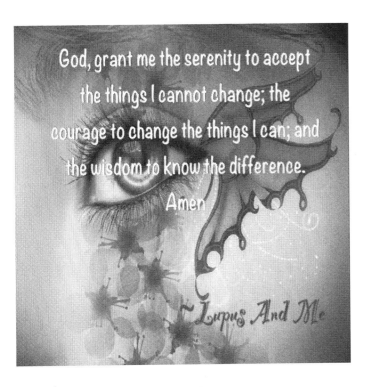

Preface

I was diagnosed with Lupus 20 years ago, after I had Chemo and radiation for uterine cancer just after the premature birth of my youngest son. At that time, internet was not born yet, so we went to the library to do research--hard to imagine nowadays! I have no thyroid anymore, as it was removed in 2009 for thyroid cancer. I have been on every regimen for lupus that there is--including plasmapereisis and IVIG--except Benlysta. I have only one kidney--born that way--and I have stage 2 nephritis. I am on cellcept, plaquenil, and prednisone for the lupus. I have been on prednisone daily for over 10 years.

As a patient with autoimmune illness (Lupus, Sjogren's, Rheumatoid Arthritis, Polymyositis, Raynaud's Syndrome, Antiphospholipid Syndrome, Celiac Disease), and nurse practitioner, I know firsthand the frustration and lack of control that these bring into our lives. Our disorders may flare at any time, may cause pain, damage and destruction to our organs, and may lead to disability, even death. That is a lot to swallow! Lupus patients often refer to this disease as "The Wolf" because of its name. But it is also a perfect visual of the characteristics that this disease holds. As with Red Riding Hood, you are never completely out of the woods and safe. Everyday issues that most people don't have to think about become magnified for us. With every slurred word...with every twinge of pain or numbness...with every rapid or slowed heart rate or indigestion, we wonder...is that the wolf lurking and licking at my heels? These feelings of having our control taken away, can lead to depression and a sense of isolation.

It is exactly for this reason that I started my Facebook page Lupus and Me, on May 31, 2012. I was in the middle of a horrible flare, and was very down, in excruciating pain, and I knew that if I was feeling this way, there were countless others in the same boat. I knew that by offering a hand in support, and having others do the same, that this would provide validation, information, laughter, and an end to the desperate feelings of loneliness many of us experience with disorders that few understand—even in the medical field. My world is different from everyone else's—it is different from what I have ever imagined for my life. I am never on solid ground—like the tectonic plates, it is always shifting beneath my feet. There is no cure for lupus. If the labs become good, it doesn't mean I am cured or had a misdiagnosis...it just means the wolf is caged, for only a brief period of time, and she will be back.

I live in Northwestern Pennsylvania, with my wonderful partner (a Certified Advanced Rolfer), of 13+ years, our 3 little dogs, and 3 children (24, 22, 20). As a family nurse practitioner, I treat many patients with Lupus and other autoimmune disorders. This is my first in a series of books on Lupus, how to live well with chronic autoimmune illness. I will also be publishing a series on overcoming childhood and relationship sexual/physical abuse.

I have recently made a job change, (I lost my previous job because of being very sick with lupus crisis/flare), working for my own wonderful physician. The flare has finally subsided after 9 months, and a recent 2 week hospital stay with massive doses of steroids. I still have a moon face, but it is fading slowly! I have chronic progressive lupus with constant low level flares (I like to call it grumbling lupus, lol), interspersed with Mega flares! I do not have health insurance for the first time in years..a bit interesting…and scary at times. I have faith that it will all work out!

Writing this book was the start on my legacy to help people learn to adapt to life in a positive way, and also to raise awareness for lupus and other chronic conditions. I believe that we are all able to grow and learn, and find joy--we just need someone to lift us up so that we see the possibility. That is what I am here for--to lift you all up, my lovelies, encouraging you to grow, find validation, gratitude, and joy, despite living with chronic illness. Never give up!

This book is my first in a series about living well with autoimmune disorders, and is geared toward providing actions that we *can* do, so that we can take back some control in our lives. This is our journey together, my lovelies.

Namaste & Blessings,

~Jenn

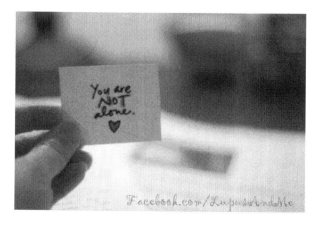

Table of Contents

Chapter 1: Autoimmune Disorders

Let food be thy medicine, and medicine be thy food.
~Hippocrates 460-377 BC

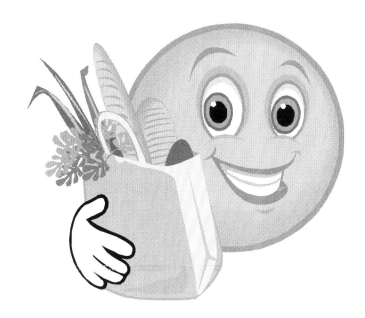

Some Statistics

Scientists worldwide puzzle over an alarming and unexplained rise in the rates of autoimmune disease. Yet the media remain quiet on this crisis.

According to American Autoimmune Related Diseases Association statistics, 50 million Americans suffer from autoimmune diseases, 75% of which are women, and the occurrences of many of the diseases are increasing. That statistic blew me away!

Autoimmune disorders are known to affect people belonging to various age groups and both genders. But certain groups are more vulnerable than others. For example, women are more prone to developing autoimmune disorders than men. Genetic predisposition may also be responsible for autoimmune diseases in members of the same family. Environmental factors such as certain chemical solvents, food allergens and other bacterial or viral presence in the air, are also known to induce autoimmune disorders.

Dr. Fred Miller, Director of the Environmental Autoimmunity Group at the National Institute of Environmental Health Sciences, says that the prevalence rates for some of these illnesses are rising for what must largely be environmental reasons. He says, "Our gene sequences aren't changing fast enough to account for the increase. Yet our environment is-- we've got 80,000 chemicals approved for use in commerce, but we know very little about their immune effects." Dr. Miller adds,

"Our lifestyles are also different than they were a few decades ago, and we're eating more processed food."

Writing in the July/August 2011 issue of Arthritis Today, rheumatologist and researcher Esther M. Sternberg, M.D., writes, "In any complex disease, the tendency to develop inflammation comes from genes, but whether it's arthritis, multiple sclerosis or something else, depends on such environmental factors as bacteria, viruses, chemicals or foreign proteins.

"In addition, there is a 'dose effect' of genes--if you inherit many autoimmune genes, you will be more likely to get an autoimmune disease, regardless of environmental exposures. If you inherit very few, then environmental factors--from chemical exposure to major stress--become more important." Dr. Sternberg points out, "The genes load the gun and the environment pulls the trigger." The good news, she suggests, is that we can do something about our environment--avoid irritants like smoke and pesticides, minimize infections with hand washing, and learn ways to cope with stress.

A combination of genetic propensity as well as environmental triggers tends to induce rapid development of autoimmune diseases. Dr Barbara Griffith, Vital health Inc founder, NMD, attributes the rising cases of autoimmune diseases to undesirable ingredients found in readymade foods found at a typical American supermarket. She adds that a poor diet and the inherently stressful lifestyles of modern America have contributed to the increase in autoimmune diseases in the US.

President and Director of the American Autoimmune Related Disease Association (AARDA), Dr Lydia Ladd suggests that the rising prevalence of autoimmune disorders can be traced more to environmental triggers such poor diets and lifestyle choices than genetic factors only. She attributes this to the fact that genetic predispositions take a long time to develop.

How do you minimize your chances of developing autoimmune disorders, and remain as healthy as possible if you already have an autoimmune disease?

- You can opt to incorporate the following lifestyle and diet changes in this book.
- Minimize the consumption of fatty, sugary and heavy foods that overload your body systems and release a constant dose of sugar into your bloodstream.
- Learn the art of relaxation with yoga, meditation techniques (will cover these in the next book). This calms down the body which can otherwise exist in a state of comparative alarm and unrest.
- Focus on consumption of important vitamins and minerals such as zinc, B-12, vitamin D, magnesium, and more, which are essential for the body.

A Little Science

Normally the immune system's white blood cells help protect the body from harmful substances, called antigens. Examples of antigens include bacteria, viruses, toxins, cancer cells, and blood or tissues from another person or species. The immune system produces antibodies that destroy these harmful substances.

In patients with an autoimmune disorder, the immune system can't tell the difference between healthy body tissue and antigens. The result is an immune response that destroys normal body tissues. This response is a hypersensitivity reaction similar to the response in allergic conditions, and causes chronic inflammation. In allergies, the immune system reacts to an outside substance that it normally would ignore. With autoimmune disorders, the immune system reacts to normal body tissues that it would normally ignore.

An autoimmune disorder may result in:

- The destruction of one or more types of body tissue
- Abnormal growth of an organ
- Changes in organ function

An autoimmune disorder may affect one or more organ or tissue types. Organs and tissues commonly affected by autoimmune disorders include:

- Blood vessels
- Connective tissues
- Heart
- Kidneys
- Brain and nervous system
- Gastrointestinal system
- Endocrine glands such as the thyroid or pancreas

- Joints
- Muscles
- Red blood cells
- Skin

A person may have more than one autoimmune disorder at the same time. Examples of autoimmune (or autoimmune-related) disorders include:

Systemic Lupus Erythematosus (SLE)-- Lupus is an autoimmune disease that can affect various parts of the body, including the skin, joints, heart, lungs, blood, kidneys and brain. Normally the body's immune system makes proteins called antibodies, to protect the body against viruses, bacteria, and other foreign materials. These foreign materials are called antigens. In an autoimmune disorder like lupus, the immune system cannot tell the difference between foreign substances and its own cells and tissues. The immune system then makes antibodies directed against itself. These antibodies -- called "auto-antibodies" (auto means 'self') -- cause inflammation, pain and damage in various parts of the body.

Celiac Disease - sprue (gluten-sensitive enteropathy)- Celiac disease is a condition that damages the lining of the small intestine and prevents it from absorbing parts of food that are important for staying healthy. The damage is due to a reaction to eating gluten, which is found in wheat, barley, rye, and possibly oats.

Multiple Sclerosis-- Multiple sclerosis is an autoimmune disease that affects the brain and spinal cord (central nervous system). MS is caused by damage to the myelin sheath, the protective covering that surrounds nerve cells. When this nerve covering is damaged, nerve signals slow down or stop.

Rheumatoid Arthritis-- A chronic autoimmune disease that is characterized especially by pain, stiffness, inflammation, swelling, and destruction of joints.

Sjogren's Syndrome-- Sjogren's syndrome is an autoimmune disease that occurs when a person's immune system attacks and destroys their moisture-producing glands. The glands affected include the person's tear and salivary glands, although their bowel, lungs and additional organs may sometimes also be affected.

Fibromyalgia--Fibromyalgia syndrome (FMS), a disorder characterized by pain or hypersensitivity in the muscles, ligaments, and tendons of the body, affects 2-4 percent of women in the general population. Up to 25 percent of women with RA, lupus, and Crohn's disease meet the American College of Rheumatology diagnostic criteria for FMS, which usually strikes women between the ages of 20 and 40. Symptoms include widespread, chronic pain, and pain sensitivity around the body. People with FMS may also suffer from fatigue, sleep disturbances, depression, anxiety, difficulty concentrating, and memory problems. Other symptoms can include migraine headaches, abdominal pain, bloating, or alternating constipation and diarrhea, and temporomandibular (TMJ) jaw pain.

The Role of Environmental Toxins

Simply put, autoimmune diseases are conditions where the body's immune system attacks its own tissues rather than a foreign molecule like bacteria. This happens when something confuses the immune system. Increasingly, that "something" appears to be the enormous load of environmental toxins to which we are all exposed. What causes the immune system to no longer tell the difference between healthy body tissues and antigens is unknown. One theory is that some microorganisms (such as bacteria or viruses) or drugs may trigger some of these changes, especially in people who have genes that make them more likely to get autoimmune disorders.

Another consideration is the continued exposure to heavy metals and environmental pollution that overload the immune system. On a daily basis, we battle with pesticides, herbicides, chemical fertilizers, industrial wastes, cigarette smoke, and automobile exhaust. Our air, water, and food (in particular) are full of toxic substances. There is no doubt that these toxins play a role in immune dysfunction. Even substances considered by most people as safe impair immune function. Sugar consumption in all forms (glucose, fructose, and sucrose) will impair the ability of white cells to destroy biological agents. This effect begins within a half hour of consumption and lasts for 5 hours. After 2 hours, immune function is reduced by 50%.

Oxidative stress plays a role in autoimmune diseases. It can be compared to a piece of metal rusting and results from the action of damaging molecules (ie, free radicals), which are a natural byproduct of the body's metabolism. The electrically charged free radicals attack healthy cells, causing them to lose their structure and function and eventually destroying them. Free radicals are not only produced by our bodies, but are also ingested from toxins and pollution in the air we breathe.

Chapter 2: The Environment, Autoimmunity, Inflammation, and Nutrition

"The doctor of the future will give no medication, but will interest his patients in the care of the human frame, diet and in the cause and prevention of disease." - Thomas A Edison

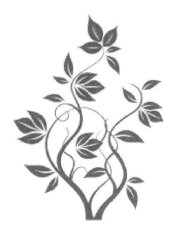

The incidence of autoimmune disease has tripled in the last few decades. In fact, it affects more women than heart disease and breast cancer combined. But autoimmune disease isn't just one condition.

We are constantly exposed to astounding amounts of pollution. Over 80,000 chemicals have been introduced into our society since 1900, and only 550 have been tested for safety. According to the US Environmental Protection Agency (EPA), about 2.5 billion pounds of toxic chemicals are released yearly by large industrial facilities. And 6 million pounds of mercury are poured into our air every year. In fact, a recent government survey - "The National Report on Human Exposure to Environmental Chemicals" issued in July 2005 -- found an average of 148 chemicals in our bodies. And those were only the ones for which they tested.

It gets worse ...

The Environmental Working Group examined the umbilical cord blood of children just as they emerged from the womb. They found 287 industrial chemicals, including pesticides, phthalates, dioxins, flame-retardants, Teflon, and toxic metals like mercury. And this was before these infants even entered the world!

That's not to mention the toxins found in our foods and other chemicals typically found in the home, like certain cleaning agents or pest control products - all of which add to the total toxic load on our bodies.

One wonders what all of this poison is doing to our children ...

In his foreword to *The Autoimmune Epidemic,* Dr. Douglas Kerr, M.D., Ph.D., a professor at Johns Hopkins School of Medicine, says that "there is no doubt that autoimmune diseases are on the rise and our increasing environmental exposure to toxins and chemicals is fueling the risk. The research is sound. The conclusions, unassailable."

Instead, we try to shut down the immune response with powerful medications including nonsteroidal anti-inflammatory drugs like Advil and Aleve, steroids like prednisone, anti-cancer drugs like methotrexate, and new drugs like Enbrel and Remicade that block the effects of a powerful inflammatory molecule called TNF alpha. Yes, they are powerful drugs, and we need to take them to keep our illnesses in check, but we also need to understand how they work so that we can keep our bodies in the best condition possible.

These new drugs shut down your immune system so powerfully that they increase your risk of cancer or life-threatening infections. And they have frequent and serious side effects and often give only partial relief. These drugs may be lifesaving for some in the short run -- but in the long run they do not address the root causes. The fact that environmental toxins are a major cause of autoimmune disease is clear. Yet conventional medicine doesn't always take that into account when treating autoimmune conditions. Much more research is needed in this area. At this point, we are only really treating the symptoms of autoimmune illness—with powerful drugs that stop our immune systems from attacking our own tissues—like taking an antihistamine for allergies—but we are still not addressing the underlying issues.

People with lupus are at a significantly increased risk of developing coronary artery disease (CAD). One study found that women between the ages of 35 and 44 who had lupus were 50-times more likely to have a heart attack than similar aged women without lupus (Manzi, 1997). Additionally, heart disease is actually one of the most common causes of death for people with lupus .This increased heart disease risk in people with lupus is caused by a several different factors (Kahlenberg, 2011), including:

1. Lupus-mediated inflammation can directly damage the endothelium, the lining of blood vessels, ultimately leading to atherosclerosis.
2. Type 2 diabetes, high blood pressure, and high cholesterol, are more likely to be present in people with lupus, all of which make the risk of heart disease greater.
3. People with lupus are often less active because of various symptoms such as fatigue, joint pain and muscle pain. A low degree of activity is associated with unhealthy weight gain and high blood pressure, both of which are risk factors of heart disease.

Leaking Gut?

Autoimmune diseases arise from an inappropriate response of the immune system to tissues in the body. The immune system identifies bodily tissues (myelin in the case of MS, joints in the case of lupus, and rheumatoid arthritis, etc.) as foreign invaders and seeks to destroy them. Food proteins can trigger the immune system to attack the self through a process called molecular mimicry. In molecular mimicry, the body sees food proteins, which have leaked through the gut (leaky gut syndrome) into the bloodstream as foreign invaders.

Those food proteins mimic bodily proteins, and so the immune system is unable to differentiate the two, and so attacks both. That is how foods can trigger symptoms in autoimmune disease. Take out the trigger foods and you have not cured your disease, but you have prevented one pathway by which symptoms occur.

There are six food triggers that tend to be common among people with autoimmune disease. But which foods trigger symptoms is idiosyncratic and varies greatly from person to person. It is imperative that you be your own detective and experiment until you find all your trigger foods. For me, it took about 4 months to identify all my trigger foods.

The six most common trigger foods are gluten, dairy, eggs, yeast, and legumes (peanuts, cashews, peas, and anything with the word bean in it), and nightshades (potatoes, peppers, eggplant). Know also that many people who react to gluten will also usually react to other grains. If you find you react to gluten, then you should also immediately suspect all other grains, including certified gluten-free oats, corn, and rice to name a few.

Heal Your Gut
Leaky Gut Syndrome is a common health disorder in which the

intestinal tract is more permeable or more porous than normal. Toxins which should naturally be repelled and eliminated leak through small openings in the lining of the intestines into the bloodstream. Leaky Gut Syndrome can cause food allergies because of the release of toxins from the gut which promotes inflammation and is associated with poor absorption of nutrients leading to some nutritional deficiencies.

If you have some of the following symptoms you could be experiencing Leaky Gut Syndrome:

- Abdominal pain
- Asthma
- Chronic joint and muscle pain
- Confusion or foggy thinking
- Mood swings & nervousness
- Recurrent vaginal infections and bladder infections
- Skin rashes such as eczema
- Bloating and gas, alternating constipation with diarrhea (usually referred to as IBS)

Some causes of Leaky Gut Syndrome are:

- Prescription antibiotic use
- Alcohol and caffeine consumption
- Chemicals in fermented and processed foods (dyes, preservatives, peroxidized fats)
- Enzyme deficiencies (e.g. celiac disease, lactase deficiency causing lactose intolerance)
- NSAIDS (non-steroidal anti-inflammatory drugs) like ibuprofen

- Prescription corticosteroids (e.g. prednisone)
- High refined carbohydrate diet (sugary foods, soft drinks and white bread)
- Prescription hormones

There is help. Leaky Gut Syndrome can be reversed by a change in diet. Eliminating sugar, white flour products, gluten, dairy products, fatty foods, caffeine products, alcohol and increasing fiber intake can combat the effects of Leaky Gut Syndrome.

When left undiagnosed or untreated, Leaky Gut Syndrome is associated with autoimmune diseases, such as lupus, rheumatoid arthritis, multiple sclerosis, fibromyalgia, chronic fatigue syndrome, Sjogren's syndrome, thyroiditis, vasculitis, Crohn's disease, ulcerative colitis, urticaria (hives), diabetes and Raynaud's disease.

How to Reverse Leaky Gut:

Food proteins that cannot cross the gut lining are unlikely to cause symptoms, so your first order of business is to heal your gut. You do this by avoiding things that irritate the gut, and by doing things that promote gut healing.

1. Avoid damaging the gut:

a. Ibuprofen and other NSAIDs

b. Antacids like TUMS and Zantac

c. Caffeine

d. Alcohol

e. Spices like chili powder, cayenne, paprika

f. Vinegar

g. Gluten

h. Antibiotics

2. Promote healing the gut:

a. Eat ½ to 1 pound of salmon per week

b. Drink Kefir and/or take a probiotic every day (Pearls, Culturelle, Reuteri, Jarrow, Renew Life, and Garden of Life are good brands.)

c. Consume homemade bone as several times per week. Either have it as a soup, or drink it as a warm drink with meals.(see Next Chapter)

Avoid Trigger Foods

Take gluten, dairy, yeast, eggs, legumes, and nightshades out of your diet. Either take them all out at once, or take gluten out one week, then dairy the next week, then yeast and legumes the following week, then nightshades the next.

Keep a detailed food diary every day and write down absolutely everything you ingest, along with any symptoms you are having. After a food has been out of your diet for at least a week, try adding it back in (add back only one food at a time) and record how you feel.

If you find that you react to gluten, you will want to take out all other grains as well to see if you react to them. Some people will know immediately that a food is a trigger food.. I didn't even add it back in to see what would happen. It was just that plain to me.

For other people, it may take a few months, or maybe even as much as a year to see results

Sleep

It is critical that you get enough sleep and enough rest. Rest means don't overdo it at work, don't exercise too much, and take some time in the midafternoon to get off your feet, whether to have a nap or just a cup of tea. Sleep means get 8-10 hours of sleep each night. Be in bed by 9 or 10 pm. Start dimming the lights as soon as it gets dark outside, and no electronics after about 7 or 8 pm. Make your bedroom pitch black (so you can't see your hand in front of your face) by removing nightlights, using blackout curtains/shades, and putting pieces of felt over clocks or other light-emitting electronics. If you have trouble falling asleep the darkness strategies mentioned should help considerably. Also try Epsom salt baths before bed.

Inflammation

Inflammation is necessary for life. Inflammation allows us to fight injury and infection. However, persistent inflammation caused by an imbalance of pro-inflammatory and anti-inflammatory chemicals leads to constant inflammation and chronic illness. Classic inflammation causes pain and resolves when wounds heal and infection is cured. Silent inflammation is not noticed until it begins to slowly damage the body's organs and cells.

Inflammation is one of the key components of most autoimmune disease. Researchers have found that diets high in refined starches, sugar, saturated fats and trans-fats actually enhance the body's inflammatory response. On the flip side, diets high in anti-inflammatory and anti-oxidant foods can decrease inflammation. These foods include fruits, vegetables, whole grains, nuts and seeds, legumes, olive oil, fish and fish oils, avocado, flax seed oil, dark chocolate, tea, spices and moderate amounts of red wine. A diet rich in these foods is healthy for anyone and vital for someone suffering from an autoimmune disease. Also, unlike many supplements, we already know that this kind of diet is beneficial and do not have to worry about dosing and medication interactions.

Anti-Inflammatory Drugs

Chronic disease, particularly autoimmune disease, is often treated with anti-inflammatory drugs. Examples of these medications include ibuprofen, prednisone, Vioxx and others. While these drugs are effective at reducing inflammation and offer numerous short-term benefits, they prevent the natural inflammatory processes that contribute to wellness. Lifelong use of anti-inflammatory compounds has many potential drawbacks including immune suppression, osteoporosis, heart disease, heart attacks and death.

Writing in his book *Toxic Fat,* Barry Sears writes that it's estimated that more people in America die each year from taking the correct dose of anti-inflammatory drugs than die from AIDS.

Eicosanoids

In 1982 the Nobel Prize was awarded to three researchers for their discovery that hormones known as eicosanoids contribute to chronic disease. These hormones include a good chemical that helps cells rejuvenate and a bad chemical that promotes cellular destruction. Because both types of processes are needed by the body, the eicosanoids must be in balance. When there's a shift toward increased production of bad eicosanoids, chronic inflammation and chronic disease develop.

Diet and Eicosanoids

All eicosanoids are derived from dietary fat in the form of essential fatty acids. The three essential fatty acids that produce eicosanoids include dihomo-gamma-linoleic acid (DGLA), arachidonic acid (AA), and eicosapentoenoic acid (EPA). DGLA and AA are omega-3 fatty acids, and EPA is an omega-3 fatty found, primarily found in fish oil. EPA and DGLA promote cellular rejuvenation, whereas the bad eicosanoid AA accelerates cellular destruction, aging, inflammation, and disease.

With a proper balance of these three fatty acids, the immune system can fight injury and infection with classic inflammation. Without this balance, chronic, toxic inflammation persists. One of its first signs is abdominal obesity. Other signs include joint inflammation, allergic reactions, metabolic syndrome, hormone imbalance, and autoimmune disease.

Fifty years ago, fatty acids in our food supply were in balance. Today, due to hybridization techniques, a move away from fish and fish oils, and increased consumption of processed foods, the western diet is in serious imbalance.

References:

Manzi, S., et al., Age-specific incidence rates of myocardial infarction and angina in women with systemic lupus erythematosus: comparison with the Framingham Study. American journal of epidemiology, 1997.

Kahlenberg, J.M. and M.J. Kaplan, The interplay of inflammation and cardiovascular disease in systemic lupus erythematosus. Arthritis research & therapy, 2011.

Sears, Barry, *Toxic Fat, When Good Fat Turns Bad*, Thomas Nelson, Nashville: 2008.

Woodson Merrell, *The Source, Unleash your Natural Energy, Power Up Your Health and Feel 10 Years Younger*, Simon & Schuster, New York: 2008.

Chapter 3: Nutrition and Autoimmune Disorders

"Take care of your body. It's the only place you have to live." ~Jim Rohn

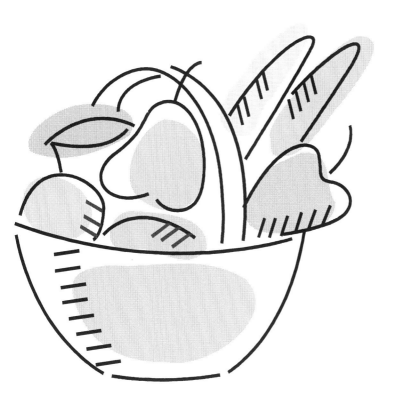

When dealing with an inflammatory disease such as Lupus or Rheumatoid Arthritis, and others, it is extremely important that you use your first line of defense, the nutrients from food, to support your body's ability to avoid and recover from flares and promote healing. There is no cure for autoimmune disease, but we can certainly maximize our health and give ourselves a much better baseline health, which will lead to faster recovery from flares, and less infections.

As with many auto immune and degenerative issues, lupus can compromise the digestive tract, making it essential that the nutrients you are eating are being absorbed. It is also necessary to determine if you have any food sensitivities and allergies, which will also affect how well you digest your food, if your body reacts to it, and therefore how you feel.

Although not often publicized, the best diet for autoimmunity and healing is ultimately the best diet for everyone, as it is derived from the unparalleled nutrition offered from fresh fruits, vegetables and whole foods, while avoiding far too common processed, fatty, refined foods, so abundant in our food stores. The simple reason this type of diet is so helpful is because it is, by nature, an anti-inflammatory diet. This diet includes simple, freshly prepared natural raw foods while eliminating fast processed foods and the 4 'white foods' including sugar, salt, flour and carbohydrates.

People with autoimmune disorders are also well advised to be careful when consuming nightshade vegetables such as tomatoes, potatoes, eggplants, and pepper in addition to alfalfa as these have been linked to trigger flares. It is important to note, however that people have different dietary needs and don't react the same to foods, so what may trigger one patient may not be a food trigger for another.

Nutrition for Autoimmune Disorders—Clean Eating

A low-fat, whole food diet is the diet of choice if you have lupus, or any disease concerning inflammation (which is implicated in most disease). Clean eating is a vital part of good health with autoimmune disease—it is a lifestyle, not a diet. So what is clean eating? Basically, clean eating means to eat food as close to its natural state of being as possible. This is kind of like how we ate 40 years ago! So, chemicals and preservatives are a no no--as much as possible.

A person that eats clean generally practices the following:

- Eliminates refined sugar
- Cooks healthy meals
- Packs healthy meals
- Makes healthy choices when dining out
- Drinks plenty of water
- Eats 5-6 small meals per day
- Eliminates alcoholic beverages (or significantly limits it)
- Always eats breakfast

"I define clean eating as consuming whole, natural foods that have not been processed," says Diane Welland, RD, author of The Complete Idiot's Guide to Eating Clean. "It's more of a lifestyle or an approach to food instead of a diet," she adds, explaining that regular physical activity and eating small, frequent meals that are balanced with protein, fat, and carbohydrates are typically part of the approach. There are countless benefits to eating more whole, natural foods: increased energy, improved immunity, lower risk of disease, and yes, loss of a few pounds.

"Weight loss comes naturally when you cut out junk food and high-calorie processed foods," says Welland. "For this reason, you don't have to worry so much about cutting calories."

A sense of social awareness is also essential to clean eating, says Susan Kleiner, PhD, RD, owner of High Performance Nutrition, a Seattle area consulting firm, and author of "The Good Mood Diet." Kleiner defines clean eating as eating foods closer to the ground - more like the way they are picked, and as you might find them at a local farmers' market. "Be mindful of how you're eating and how what you eat affects the world around you," she says.

When shopping for cereal, bread and pasta, don't just look for the words "whole grain" on a food's packaging. Read ingredient lists carefully, looking for the word "whole" in front of each type of flour. Another trick for picking out clean-diet offenders: "High fructose corn syrup is a flag," says Kleiner. "The fact that it's added means the food is highly processed."

A processed food is one that has been taken apart and put back together in order to create properties that may not occur naturally, or those that have to be replaced, says Kleiner, explaining that chemicals - some not found in nature - are often used in the process.

Grains are a good example. Like the name implies, whole grains contain an entire grain kernel (bran, germ and endosperm), while refined grains have been milled, a process that strips out bran and germ, along with fiber, iron and B vitamins. This process gives the grains a finer texture and a longer shelf life (think soft, fluffy white bread that lasts for weeks in the fridge). Refined grains are typically enriched, meaning iron and B vitamins, such as thiamin, riboflavin, folic acid and niacin, are removed and then added back after milling, but fiber is left out.

Keep in mind that many foods have to be processed in some way in order to make them edible, so the idea is to pick the least processed variety, says Kleiner. Cereal oats are a good example. While we can't eat them unprocessed, we can select steel-cut oatmeal over oat flakes, or oat flakes over oat-based cereal with added coloring, flavoring and fun-shaped marshmallows.

When food additives and preservatives are considered, you probably think of a chemical compound spelled with no fewer than 16 characters - and one that you wouldn't dare try to pronounce. But other extras sound much more benign - sugar and salt, for example, which are often added to food in excess to boost flavor or extend shelf life.

The key to finding the "cleanest" possible foods is asking yourself a few questions: Are the ingredients natural or artificial? Are all the ingredients really necessary? Can I buy this product minus the offending ingredient, and will that absence affect the integrity of the food?

Take salt, for example. It's used as a preservative in cheese, and is essential to the cheese-making process, says Welland. Adding salt to canned vegetables, on the other hand, is unnecessary, as it isn't part of the production process and the veggies can be purchased either fresh or frozen without salt.

Another example is yogurt. Yogurt is produced by culturing milk, but fruit-flavored yogurt also have other things added to it including sugar, says Welland. Consider how easily fresh fruit can be stirred into plain yogurt for a lower sugar (and calorie) option, she says.

And what about the chemical-sounding additives? Only a few are natural and safe to consume regularly, says Kleiner. Citric acid (vitamin C, a natural antioxidant), vitamin E (an antioxidant that appears as tocopherols on food labels), and carotene (used to boost color) are commonly used as preservatives.

With excess sugar consumption linked to cancer, diabetes and heart disease, numerous white sugar alternatives have made their way onto grocery store shelves. Maple sugar, agave nectar and evaporated cane sugars, like secant, have stronger flavors than white sugar, which means you can get the same sweetness with fewer calories. Less-refined varieties of sugar come with a higher price tag, which Kleiner sees as something positive. "When sugar is more expensive, you don't treat it as nonchalantly. You think twice about using it and stop taking it for granted."

Still, sugar is sugar, no matter what its form, and moderation is key. A bonus that comes with cutting back on added sugar: "When you start taking out a lot of sugar and salt, you are retraining your taste buds and you tend to appreciate the natural sweet tastes of foods like beets and peas, or maybe the earthiness of a mushroom," Kleiner says.

When it comes to fat, the hydrogenated oils typically found in empty calorie foods like doughnuts, candy, and cookies are the biggest offenders in a clean diet. Highly engineered fats, like the trans fat in man-made oils, are worse at promoting heart disease than natural fats, like lard, says Kleiner. According to Kleiner, a food label reading zero grams of trans fat - which is allowed for any item that contains less than half a gram per serving - can be misleading. Kleiner's general rule: "If it has hydrogenated oil in it, don't buy it. It's also a sign that it's a highly processed food. Go for something less processed."

"Clean eating doesn't mean vegetarian. It means choosing meat from grass- or vegetarian-fed (grass and grain-fed) animals," says Kleiner. Animal feed can be filled with antibiotics, hormones, fertilizers and chemicals. Instead, turn to pasture-fed or free-range animals, which have more nutritiously rich meat and a healthier fatty acid composition. Meat that comes from pasture-fed animals is naturally lower in saturated fat and contributes less to heart disease risk.

You can also have a clean diet without meat. Beans, legumes, nuts and nut butters are big in the clean-eating realm. They provide crunch, texture, protein and a concentrated source of calories, says Welland.

"Diets abundant in fruits and veggies - whether grown organically or conventionally - are healthier than diets without them," say Kleiner. A significant body of research shows the link between fruit and vegetable consumption and lower incidences of cardiovascular disease, stroke and cancer, and improved gastrointestinal and optical health. Additionally, in a review of 97 studies that compared the nutritional composition of organic versus conventional foods, researchers found that organic fruits, vegetables, and grains were 25 percent more nutrient-dense than conventional food. Organic produce and grains contain higher levels of 8 out of 10 nutrients studied, according to the report published by The Organic Center.

If you've purchased conventional fruits and vegetables, scrub them thoroughly, using a produce detergent to remove wax, or peel off the skin before eating, suggests Kleiner.

Water, unsweetened tea, milk, and 100 percent fruit juice mixed with water or seltzer are standard beverages for clean eaters, but caffeine isn't out of the question. Still, experts are on the fence about where it falls in a clean diet. Welland points out that many beverages that are high in caffeine, like soft drinks, also tend to be high in sugar. On the other hand, coffee and tea are natural products that are high in antioxidants. Welland's general rule: If you're sensitive to caffeine, limit your consumption or cut it out of your diet. If you don't have a strong reaction, caffeine is fine in small amounts, she says.

Kleiner recommends drinking no more than two caffeinated drinks per day and avoiding those beverages after noontime.

"If you feel like you need caffeine later in the day, you probably should to take another look at the way you're living your life," she says. "Are you dehydrated? Do you need to be more active? Do you need more sleep? Do you have too much stress in your life?"

If you can't get by without a boost, Kleiner suggests reaching for tea instead of coffee in the afternoon. "Tea is much lower in caffeine, less acidic, and less harsh on the body, she says.

If there's one downside to clean eating it's the extra time it takes to shop for and prepare your meals - but for many, it's time well spent. "You have to prioritize," says Welland. "Ask yourself, 'Do I want more time or a healthy meal, better health, and to feel good?'"

With a little planning and creativity, Welland says, cooking clean meals can become easier than playing around with combinations of prepared or microwave-ready foods. She likes to start with basic ingredients and think of ways to bring out the natural flavors in food - drizzling roasted sweet potatoes with a little maple syrup, or stirring cilantro and salsa into a side of black beans, for example. Welland dresses up veggies by experimenting with simple spice blends, tinkering with combinations of chili powder, cumin, coriander, basil and garlic.

Snacks and meals should be balanced with protein, fat, and carbohydrates and are generally not overly done in any one area. For example, instead of grabbing an apple for a snack, have an apple with peanut butter, or try red bell pepper slices with hummus, suggests Welland.

Oh No, Not Another Diet!

So, you are ready to start getting healthier? I know that personally, I tend to go all out on something new, and then decide I cannot continue it. This is not a diet—it is a lifestyle, and will require some getting used to, so be easy on yourself! I recommend that you start with trying to eat clean for one meal a day—and see how you feel after 1 week! One week is doable for anything, right?

Not only will it decrease your joint pain, reduce strain on the kidneys, spleen and other organs, it will also lower your blood pressure and cholesterol levels and reduce the risk of heart attack. Another added benefit is it will also support weight loss, which many autoimmune sufferers write to me about, as a consequence of steroid side effects.

We tell ourselves that we cannot eat healthy because "it costs too much." This is simply not true...Using a crockpot and a few fresh veggies along with fresh meat can provide several meals, is tastier, and much more fulfilling, and far cheaper than a frozen dinner!

I know with lupus and other chronic illnesses, fatigue is a big part of life. So, the idea of cooking something makes us go, "no way is that happening." I highly recommend a crockpot—it is very easy to whip up tasty meals that are easy on the budget, with little effort.

It is also important to note that everyone has their own view of what they consider "eating clean". Some people will be stricter than others depending on their goals (which is fine). You need to find out what works for you and your body. **As long as you are making healthier choices for you and your family - you are moving in the right direction.**

Eating clean can be a major transition for a majority of people due to addictions to sugar, white bread, and fast food. It takes discipline in order to make eating clean a habit but it is possible and has so many long-term health benefits.

Another point I would like to share is that you should **NOT EXPECT PERFECTION!** You'll never have a "perfect diet" or a "perfect body". I am still learning more about clean eating...it was overwhelming at first, but, over time, you will figure out the approach that best fits your budget and time constraints.

Jenn's Eating Clean-Simplified:

- Eat only whole foods. That means eating oats and blueberries rather than a blueberry muffin. When you eat packaged foods, only buy brands that contain "real food" ingredients--ingredients you easily recognize, can pronounce, and would use to make a "from scratch" version in your own kitchen. If a food contains even one ingredient that makes you think "huh?" skip it, at least during the clean eating challenge.

- Drink plenty of water—2-3 liters daily. NOTE: Do not do this if you have kidney disease or congestive heart failure—please check with your physician first.

- Consume bone broth daily (See next chapter).

- Eat plenty of fruits and vegetables. Choose fresh, unprocessed foods over canned or processed products. Clean eating enthusiasts believe that we were meant to survive on fresh fruits and vegetables and that processing them reduces their nutritional value and fiber content and adds salt, fat, sugar and chemicals. Choose fruit instead of fruit juice and if you must pick a processed vegetable, frozen is always better than canned.

- Include meats, however; "whole" meats that you have chosen straight from the butcher or prepared yourself. You would be very surprised to find out what is actually in ground turkey.

- Eliminate refined sugar. Refined sugar provides nothing but calories. Other sweeteners can be used, but with all the good foods you add to your diet, refined sugar really has very little place in the eating clean plan.

- Enjoy whole grains - these are grains that are still complete and haven't been broken down in any form. Examples include: brown rice, whole wheat and other whole grains. You will have to get used to reading over food labels. Just because a product says its "whole grain" does not mean it is. It also does not mean they have not added a bunch of other ingredients as well.

- Eat fewer ingredients - try not to purchase items with more than 4-6 ingredients in the ingredient list. Also, be sure you recognize every ingredient. If you can't pronounce it, you probably shouldn't put it in your body. Delicious, healthy food doesn't have to contain a lot of ingredients. Keep your meal ingredients to a minimum— just be sure to include a source of whole grains, lean protein and healthy fat at each meal. For example, veggies and shrimp stir fried in sesame oil over a bed of brown rice seems restaurant quality but can be whipped up faster than takeout.

- Eat slower- Put your fork or spoon down between every bite, and focus on the flavors and textures of your food.

- Eat five or six small meals a day. By eating smaller meals throughout the day you can help rev up your metabolism and reduce the chance that you'll eat some chips rather than that whole grain cracker with nut butter and strawberries. You never get so hungry on this plan that you'll feel deprived or feel the need to cheat.

- Eat on a regular schedule. Try not to let more than about 4 hours go by between meals or snacks. Steady meal timing helps regulate your digestive system, blood sugar and insulin levels, and appetite.

- Avoid sodas and high calorie, sugary drinks. Follow the tenant of clean eating that aims to remove added sugars from the diet. Choose water or tea for your beverages, or juice your own fruits and vegetables and enjoy them without added sugars or preservatives.

Most importantly, this diet will reduce the number of antigen-antibodies in your body, a primary factor that causes lupus and autoimmune flares. Many people are now aware of the great health benefits derived from Omega 3. The primary benefit concerns the fact that these essential fatty acids act as an anti-inflammatory, exactly what we need if we have lupus. Therefore, with reduced inflammation comes reduced pain and increased mobility.

Because our common food intake doesn't provide enough of these healthy fats, it is extremely wise (especially if you have lupus) to supplement with them. Flaxseed oil is a popular source of Omega 3, however recently there is evidence that your best source of omega 3 comes from fish oil, in particular krill oil. Of course, eating a diet rich with Omega 3 is important, and the most common source of EFA's is from salmon, and other cold-water fish such as tuna. Other sources include avocados, spinach, and mustard greens.

References:

Kleiner, Susan. *The Good Mood Diet.* Springboard Press: 2007

Welland, Diane. *The Complete Idiots Guide to Eating Clean.* Alpha: 2008.

Chapter 4: The Benefits of Bone Broth

One should eat to live, not live to eat" -Benjamin Franklin

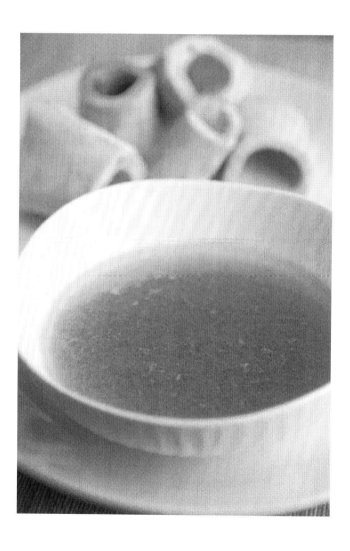

"Good broth will resurrect the dead," says a South American proverb. Said Escoffier, "Indeed, stock is everything in cooking. Without it, nothing can be done."

Bone broth is commonly used in the making of high quality restaurant soups, though it is seldom made in the average modern American household. It seemed to fall out of favor as "fast food" became more popular, but as both a flavorful and valuable nutritional food it is well worth making, especially in the winter season.

The broth is easy to make, with the main drawback being that it takes time to cook. Once made, it can be consumed plain as a snack or quick meal, or used as the base for a more complex soup by adding steamed or sautéed vegetables, meat, and/or beans. It may also be used as a base for sauces or added in place of water in the cooking of rice or other grains.

Major Constituents of Bones and Bone Broth

Cartilage

Cartilage is formed primarily from collagen and elastin proteins, but also contains glycosaminoglycans (GAGs), chondroitin sulfate, keratin sulfate, and hyaluronic acid. The cartilage from joints is the kind incorporated into bone broth.

Chondroitin sulfate is a structural component of cartilage and is essential in maintaining the integrity of the extracellular matrix. It also lines the blood vessels, and has been found to play a role in lowering cholesterol and the incidence of heart attacks. It is often sold as a supplement for treating joint pain associated with osteoarthritis and has been shown to improve inflammatory conditions of the gastrointestinal tract.

Studies have found shark cartilage to be useful in the treatment of joint disease and in the stimulation of immune cells, but these supplements can be very expensive. Using cartilage-rich beef knuckles, chicken feet, trachea, and ribs in a bone soup can be an effective and easily absorbable alternative. Cartilage may be useful in the treatment of:

- Arthritis
- Degenerative joint disease
- Inflammatory bowel disease
- Lowered immune function

Bone Marrow

There are two types of marrow in bones, yellow and red. At birth, all bone marrow is red, and as we age it gradually converts to the yellow type until only about half of our marrow is red. In cases of severe blood loss, the yellow marrow can change back to red marrow as needed, in order to increase blood cell production.

The yellow marrow is concentrated in the hollow interior of the middle portion of long bones, and is where lipids and fats are stored. The red marrow is found mainly in the flat bones, such as the hip bone, sternum, skull, ribs, vertebrae and scapula, and in the cancellous ("spongy") material at the proximal ends of the long bones such as the femur and humerus. Red marrow is where the myeloid stem cells and lymphoid stem cells are formed.

The red marrow is an important source of nutritional and immune support factors extracted in the cooking of bone soup. It contains myeloid stem cells which are the precursors to red blood cells, and lymphoid stem cells, the precursors to white blood cells and platelets. The red marrow produces these immature precursor cells, which later convert to mature cell outside the marrow.

- Red blood cells carry oxygen to other cells in the body
- White blood cells are essential for proper functioning of the immune system
- Platelets are important for clotting

Glycine and Proline

Glycine and proline are particularly important amino acids present in bone broth. Glycine is a simple amino acid necessary in the manufacture of other amino acids. It is a vital component in the production of heme, the part of the blood that carries oxygen. It is also involved in glucogenesis (the manufacture of glucose), supports digestion by enhancing gastric acid secretion, and is essential for wound healing. It is a precursor amino acid for glutathione and large amounts are needed for the liver to detoxify after chemical exposure.

Broths can be used in modified fasting and cleansing programs. In these situations, glycine is used for gluconeogenesis and to support phase I and II detoxification. During fasting, because little or no food or energy source is being consumed, protein tissues such as muscle often break down. With broth, glycine is consumed, which limits or prevents degeneration during the fast and is also beneficial to the detoxification process.

Proline is an amino acid essential to the structure of collagen and is therefore necessary for healthy bones, skin, ligaments, tendons and cartilage. It is found in small amounts in many foods, but vitamin C is necessary to metabolize proline into its active form. Small amounts can be manufactured by the body, but evidence shows that adequate dietary protein is necessary to maintain an optimal level of proline in the body. It has also been shown to have a beneficial effect on memory and in the prevention of depression.

Glycine and proline are needed for:

- Manufacture of glucose
- Enhancing gastric acid secretion
- Soft tissue and wound healing
- Healthy connective tissue
- Effective detoxification by the liver
- Production of plasma
- Improves hair and nails
- Re-mineralizes teeth

Collagen and Gelatin

There are at least 15 types of collagen, making up about 25% of all the protein in the body. It is present in bones, ligaments, tendons and skin (type I collagen), in cartilage (type II collagen), and in bone marrow and lymph (type III collagen, called reticulin fiber). The word collagen comes from the root "kola", meaning glue.

Basically, collagen is the same as gelatin. Collagen is the word used for its form when found in the body, and gelatin refers to the extracted collagen that is used as food.

Bone broth produces a rubbery gelatin when cooled. Most commercial gelatin products are made from animal skin and often contain MSG, but broth made from bones produces a much more nutritious gelatin that contains a wide range of minerals and amino acids.

Poor wound healing, bleeding gums, and bruising are often been attributed to vitamin C deficiency, however the problem is actually a collagen deficiency, as vitamin C is needed to synthesize collagen. Gelatin has also been found to help heal the mucus membranes of the gastrointestinal tract in cases of inflammation such as irritable bowel syndrome or in "leaky gut syndrome".

Gelatin is rich in the amino acids proline and glycine. Although it is not a complete protein itself, it provides many amino acids and therefore decreases the amount of complete protein needed by the body. Dr. N. R. Gotthoffeer spent 20 years studying gelatin and found that convalescing adults who have lost weight due to surgery, dysentery, cancer and other diseases fare much better if gelatin is added to their diet.

Studies on gelatin show that it increases the digestion and utilization of many dietary proteins such as beans, meat, milk and milk products. Collagen is helpful in:

- Soft tissue and wound healing

- Formation and repair of cartilage and bone

- Healing and coating the mucus membranes of the gastrointestinal tract

- Facilitating digestion and assimilation of proteins

Minerals

Minerals are essential to life, providing the basis for many important functions in the body. They are necessary for the development of connective tissue and bone, create electrical potential that facilitates nerve conduction, and are catalysts for enzymatic reactions. Many people in the U.S. are deficient in one or more minerals, usually due to dietary deficiencies or poor absorption. Broth offers easily absorbed extracted minerals and supports utilization of the minerals by promoting the health of the intestinal tract.

Bone is an excellent source of calcium and phosphorus, and to a lesser degree, magnesium, sodium, potassium, sulfate and fluoride. Hydrochloric acid, produced by the stomach, helps to break down food but is also necessary to extract elemental minerals from food. For this reason, when making bone broth, an acid is necessary in order to extract the minerals from the bone. This is the purpose of adding a "splash" of vinegar when making broth.

- Calcium is necessary for healthy bones, muscle contraction and relaxation, proper clotting and tissue repair, normal nerve conduction, and endocrine balance. Calcium deficiency includes symptoms of osteomalacia and osteoporosis, brittle nails, periodontal disease, muscle cramps and spasms, palpitations, depression, insomnia, and hyperactivity.

- Phosphorus is necessary for the generation of energy in the body, as it is an important ingredient of ATP. It is also a critical component of cell membranes and helps regulate intracellular pressure. A deficiency in phosphorus can lead to symptoms such as fatigue, weakness, muscle weakness, celiac disease, osteomalacia, and seizures.

- Magnesium is the most common dietary deficiency in the U.S. The mineral is involved in over 300 enzyme reactions, is a cofactor for vitamins B1 and B6, and is involved in the synthesis of proteins, fatty acids, nucleic acids and prostaglandins. Proper nerve transmission, muscle contraction and relaxation, and parathyroid gland function are dependent on magnesium.

How to Cook Bone Broth

The bones and cartilage of most meats can be used, including poultry, beef, lamb or fish. Pork bones are not generally used for making broth that is cooked for many hours and stored to be re-heated and used later, though they may be included in stew and soup recipes. Quality bones are recommended, such as those from organic meats, and natural, grass-fed beef, with the fat and most of the meat trimmed off.

Chicken carcass is a good choice as it has a high concentration of red marrow. Beef and lamb bones give a nicer broth if they have been roasted in the oven first, until browned (400 degrees F or 200 degrees C for 45-90 minutes). Though bones leftover from cooking other dishes may be used, bones specifically used for making broth may also be bought at most supermarkets.

If possible, use kitchen scissors to break the bones into smaller pieces, ideally 2-3 inches long, increasing the surface area of bone exposed to the boiling water therefore increasing the quality and nutrient value of the soup. For larger bones, your supermarket butcher will usually cut them for you.

Place the bones in a stockpot and just cover with cold water. Add a "splash", or about 2 tablespoons, of rice, wine, cider, or balsamic vinegar per quart of water or per about 2 pounds of bones. An acid such as vinegar is necessary in order to extract the minerals and nutrients from the bone into the soup. Lemon juice may be substituted for the vinegar. Garlic, onions and ginger may be added for increased flavor, as well as coarsely chopped pieces of celery, carrot, parsley and other vegetables.

Cooking and storing the broth

Heat the stock very slowly, gradually bringing to a boil, then turn heat down and simmer for at least 6 hours, removing the scum as it arises. 6 - 48 hours is an ideal cooking time for chicken bones and 12 - 72 hours for beef. If the bones are cut into smaller pieces first, this will reduce the necessary cooking time. Do not allow the broth to come to a fast boil, and if more water is needed to keep the bones covered, add only hot water, not cold or lukewarm.

Cooking in a crockpot on low setting is an easy way to cook broth for a prolonged time. Though it is not necessary to remove the surface scum that arises, doing so occasionally during the cooking process will result in a nicer tasting broth.

After simmering the bones for several hours, other vegetables may be added for the last 1-2 hours of cooking. This adds to both the flavor and nutritional value of the broth.

When finished cooking, the bones and vegetables can be removed and discarded, and the liquid strained through a colander. For a clear soup, it should be strained a second time through a hair sieve or a colander lined with cheesecloth. Parboiling and rinsing the bones before cooking and cooking on a low heat can also help produce a clear broth as it greatly reduces the amount of residue in the liquid.

The broth should be set to cool until the fat hardens on top, then remove the fat and refrigerate the broth. It will keep for about 5 days in the refrigerator, or 10 days if it is boiled again in 5 days, and can be kept for months in the freezer. Before re-heating, always remove and discard any residual fat from the top. Properly prepared broth will cool to a rubbery, jellylike consistency due to the high gelatin content of the collagen. It can be re-heated and used as a simple nutritious drink, or for a more complex soup, add steamed or sautéed vegetables, meat, and/or beans.

Emily's Bone Broth Soup Recipes:
Basic Bone Broth
Ingredients:

- 2-3 lbs soup bones (marrow, knuckle, meaty bones, or a whole chicken or turkey carcass)
- Purified water
- 1 tbsp raw, unfiltered apple cider vinegar ("ACV")

Process:

1. Add soup bones to crock pot.
2. Fill crock pot with just enough water to slightly cover the bones, if some bones are sticking out that's ok!
3. Add 1 tbsp of ACV to the crock pot, cover, turn onto low, and slow cook for 24-48 hours.
4. Turn the crock pot off and allow to cool.
5. Strain the broth through a fine mesh strainer
6. Keep in the fridge in a glass container, for up to a week. You can boil the broth after a week to kill any bacteria, in which case it will last longer. You can also keep the broth frozen in ice cube trays, and pop out a few cubes each time you desire it.
7. Heat the broth on the stove top before each use.

Winter Bone and Vegetable Soup

1-2 pounds of bones (lamb, chicken, or beef), chopped into large pieces

2 tomatoes, peeled, seeded, and halved

2 small potatoes, peeled and quartered

1 onion, peeled and quartered

3 garlic cloves, peeled

2 sticks celery, peeled and cut in half

2 carrots, peeled and cut in half

5 whole sprigs of parsley

1 tsp. black peppercorns

1-2 tablespoons balsamic vinegar

salt to taste

1. Preheat oven to 400° F
2. Rinse bones and place in a foil-lined tray.
3. Roast bones, uncovered, until brown on all sides, turning every 20 minutes.

   (Approximately 1-2 hours, depending on amount of bones.)
4. Add bones to stockpot with 1 1/2 quarts of cold water, or enough to cover the bones.
5. Slowly bring to a boil, then turn down and simmer gently
6. Add peppercorns, garlic, onions, and 2-3 teaspoons vinegar
7. Cook half-covered, for 4+ hours. Add more boiling water if necessary when simmering, in order to keep bones covered.
8. Skim surface every half hour to remove scum and impurities - do not stir though!

9. Strain, cool broth, and remove any fat that comes to the surface.

10. Prepare carrots, celery, parsley, tomatoes, and potatoes

11. Heat broth, add cut up vegetables, and simmer for 1 more hour.

Beef Bones and Greens Soup

5-6 grass-fed beef bones, plus a large marrow bone (if available)

2 c. fresh collards, chopped

2 c. fresh kale, torn into bite sized pieces

3 carrots, sliced

1/2 c. green cabbage, sliced or chopped

1 cup chopped fresh cilantro and/or parsley

2 shallot bulbs, separated and chopped

5 cloves garlic, minced

1/2-1 inch piece of ginger, minced

vinegar

Herbs and seasonings as desired:

rosemary

bay leaf

fresh sage leaves

red pepper flakes, crushed

sea salt and pepper

curry powder

Italian seasoning

tamari or soy sauce

1. Clean off bones and add to pot with enough cold water to cover bones

2. Bring slowly to a boil. Turn heat to low and add ginger, garlic, shallots, and vinegar

3. Cover and simmer for 6 hours.

4. Allow to cool, and place in refrigerator overnight for excess fat to congeal; you may want to get your hands dirty and fish out any cartilage and fat still stuck on the meat at this point.

5. On the day that you want to eat the soup, remove the pot form the refrigerator and use a large spoon to scrape off the top fat layer.

6. Place the pot back on the stove and turn to medium high heat. Add vegetables and spices.

7. Cook at a simmer until ready to serve. Remove bones before serving.

Basic Chicken Broth

1 whole free-range chicken or 2 to 3 pounds of bony chicken parts, such as necks, backs, breastbones and wings

4 quarts cold filtered water

2 tablespoons vinegar

1 large onion, coarsely chopped

2 carrots, peeled and coarsely chopped

3 celery stalks, coarsely chopped

1 bunch parsley

1. If using a whole chicken, cut off the wings, remove the neck and cut both into pieces. Remove gizzards from the cavity. If using chicken parts, cut them into several pieces.

2. Place chicken and pieces in a pot with cold water, vinegar and all vegetables except parsley.

3. Bring slowly to a boil, and remove scum that rises to the top.

4. Reduce heat, cover and simmer for 6 to 8 hours. Cooking longer will give a richer and more flavorful broth.

5. About 10 minutes before finishing cooking, add parsley.

6. Remove whole chicken or pieces with a slotted spoon, reserving the meat for other use.

7. Strain the stock into a large bowl and refrigerate until the fat rises to the top and congeals.

8. Skim off the fat and keep stock in the refrigerator or freezer for future use.

References:

Traditional bone broth in modern health and disease.

Allison Siebecker; Townsend Letter 2005.

Chapter 5: Nutrients Depleted by Medications

"Your body is a temple, but only if you treat it as one." ~Astrid Alauda

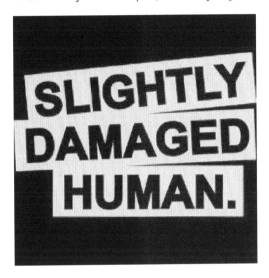

DRUG CATEGORY OF NUTRIENTS DEPLETED

ANTACIDS
All that contain aluminum or magnesium :

Calcium, Phosphorus, Chromium, Vitamin D, Iron, Zinc

ANTIBIOTICS
All

B Vitamins, Vitamin K, Calcium, Magnesium, Iron
Lactobacillus Acidophilus

Tetracycline,Doxycycline and Bactrim, Septra
Magnesium, Calcium, All B Vitamins

ANTIDIABETICS
Sulfonylureas: Glynase,Prandin,Glucotrol
Coenzyme Q10
Metformin(Glucophage)
Vitamin B12, Folic Acid, Coenzyme Q10

ANTI-INFLAMMATORIES
Aspirin
Vitamin C, Folic Acid, Potassium, Iron, Sodium
NSAIDS (All)
Folic Acid, Melatonin, Iron, Potassium
Corticosteroids(Prednisone, etc.)
Calcium, Vitamin A, Vitamin D, Potassium, Zinc, Vitamin

B 6, Vitamin C, Vitamin K, Magnesium, Folic Acid, Selenium , DHEA

BENZODIAZEPINES
Valium, Ativan
Melatonin

CARDIAC AND HYPERTENSION DRUGS
Lasix, Bumex
Calcium, Magnesium, Vitamin B1, Vitamin B6,Vitamin C, Potassium, Zinc
Hydrochlorthiazide (HCTZ), Hydrodiuril
Magnesium, Potassium, Zinc, Folic Acid, Coenzyme Q10
Dyazide, Maxide
Calcium, Folic Acid, Zinc
ACE Inhibitors
(Prinivil, Zestril, Altace etc) and ARBs (Valsartan, losartan, olmesartan, irbesartan, telmisartan, azilsartan
CoEnzyme Q10, Zinc, Vitamin B1, Phosphorus, Vitamin B1, Sodium
Clonidine, Aldomet
Coenzyme Q10, Calcium, Magnesium, Zinc
Beta-Blockers
Coenzyme Q10, Melatonin
Digoxin
Calcium, Magnesium, Phosphorous, Vitamin B1

CHOLESTEROL LOWERING DRUGS
All Statins (Lipitor, Pracachol, Zocor, etc)

Coenzyme Q10, Vitamin D

Bile Acid Binders(Cholestyramine, Colestipol)
Vitamin A, Vitamin D, Vitamin E Vitamin K, Vitamin B12,
Folic Acid, Iron, Calcium,Magnesium, Phosphorous, Zinc

FEMALE HORMONES
Birth Control Pills
Vitamins B2, Vitamin B6, Vitamin B12, Vitamin C, Folic
Acid, Magnesium, Zinc
Estrogens
Magnesium, Zinc, Vitamin B6

PSYCHIATRIC MEDICATIONS
Tricyclic Antidepressants (Amitryptaline, desipramine,
nortryptaline, doxepin, imipramine); Phenothiazines (Haloperidol,
fluphenazine, chlorpromazine)
Coenzyme Q10, Vitamin B12, Folic Acid
SSRIs and SNRIs
(Fluoxetine, paroxetine, sertraline, citalopram, escitalopram,
duloxetine, venlafaxine)
Vitamin B6, Vitamin B12, Folic Acid, Sodium, Vitamin D,
Essential Fatty Acids
Atypical Medications
(Risperidone, olanzapine, aripirazole, quetiapine, buproprion)
Coenzyme Q10, Vitamin B12, Essential Fatty Acids, Folic
Acid

RHEUMATOLOGY MEDICATIONS
Anti-Malarials
(Hydroxychloroquine, Chloroquine

Calcium, Vitamin B6, Vitamin D
Antineoplastics/Antimetabolities (methotrexate,
cyclophosphamide)

Calcium, Folic Acid, Magnesium, Potassium, Selenium,

Vitamin C, Carnitine, Choline
Immunosuppressants
(Mycophenolate, tacrolimus, azathioprine, cyclosporine)

Calcium, Magnesium, Vitamin C

ULCER MEDICATIONS
H2- Blockers
Tagamet, Pepcid, Zantac, Axid

Vitamins B12, Vitamin D, Folic Acid, Calcium, Iron, Zinc
Proton Pump Inhibitors
Prevacid, Protonix, Aciphex, Nexium

Vitamin B12, magnesium

As you can see, our medications deplete many important nutrients, which, coupled with the stress on our bodies from having chronic illness, can lead to worsening of our symptoms, and diminishes our overall health. In addition, the fatigue from the above illnesses can preclude us from always eating a completely healthy or clean diet. So, we need to take some supplements to make up for this. The quality of our supplements is extremely important.

References:

Pelton, Lavalle, Hawkins, Krinsky. Drug-Induced Nutrient Depletion Handbook. Lexi-Comp; 2nd Ed., 2001.

Pelton R Lavalle. The Nutritional Cost of Prescription Drugs. Morton Publishing Co, 2nd Ed., 2004.

Vaglini F, Fox B. The Side Effects Bible: The Dietary Solution to Unwanted Side Effects of Common Medications.Broadway, 2005.

Chapter 6: Vital Nutrients and Food Sources

"Today, more than 95% of all chronic disease is caused by food choice, toxic food ingredients, nutritional deficiencies and lack of physical exercise." ~ Mike Adams

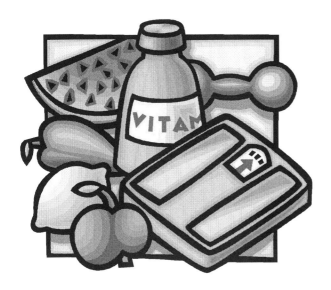

Vitamin B1 (thiamine)

Function and Effect - Required by all cells in the body to make the source of energy and fuel (ATP); plays a major role in blood sugar conversion; necessary for maintenance of nerve tissues, functions, and transmissions; maintains muscles, especially the heart; synthesizes acetylcholine (primary neurotransmitter involved in memory and thought processes); involved in the synthesis of fatty acids.

Effects of depletion/deficiency - Considered to be one of the most common nutrient deficiencies in the U.S., a Department of Agriculture study estimates that 45% of the population gets less than the RDA (Recommended Daily Allowance) of Vitamin B1. Deficiencies will appear as disorders in the cardiovascular, gastrointestinal, and neuromuscular systems. Symptoms include depression, irritability, memory loss, mental confusion, indigestion, weight loss, edema, anorexia, sore calf muscles, loss of reflexes in legs, anorexia, defective muscular coordination, muscle weakness, rapid pulse, heart palpitations, fatigue, nerve inflammation with possible sensation of pins and needles and numbness.

Dosage range - RDA 1.5 mg. daily; typical dosage range is 1.5-100 mg. daily. Therapeutic treatment doses are 200-600 mg. daily. Toxicity and overdose is unlikely (doses would have to be 2 grams or more).

Dietary sources - All animal and plant foods contain low concentrations of B1. Whole, intact cereal grains also provide

B1. Organ meats and brewer's yeast are the richest sources of B1.

Vitamin B2 (riboflavin)

Function and Effect - B2 combines with phosphoric acid becoming part of two important coenzymes that bind 100+ enzymes that act as antioxidants in the cells; facilitates metabolism of carbohydrates, proteins, and fats; assists in converting carbohydrates to ATP in the production of energy; assists in growth of healthy hair, skin, and nails; assists in reproductive process.

Effects of depletion/deficiency - deficiencies of B1 occur most often as a component of multiple nutrient deficiencies. Symptoms include soreness and burning of mouth, tongue, and lips; cracks in the corners of the mouth (chelosis); inflamed mucous membranes; itchy, dry, possibly scaly skin with eczema on the face and genitals; eyes that tear, itch, burn, are sensitive to light and tire easily. Depression and hysteria can result from long term deficiency that damages nerve tissue.

Dosage range - RDA 1.7 mg daily; typical daily dosage range is 1.2-100 mg. daily. B2 is not known to be toxic.

Dietary sources - The largest amounts of B2 are found in milk and other dairy products, and liver. Moderate amounts are in salmon and tuna, with somewhat less found in other fish; oysters; eggs; mushrooms; dark green vegetables; avocados.

Vitamin B3 (niacin)

Function and Effect - Niacin is a part of two coenzymes that are involved in over 200 reactions in the metabolism of carbohydrates, amino acids, and fatty acids. It is critical to maintaining the function of every cell in the body. B3 also acts as an antioxidant; reduces LDL cholesterol and triglycerides while raising HDL cholesterol; helps cells in being sensitive to insulin; has anti-anxiety properties.

Effects of depletion/deficiency - dermatitis, dementia, diarrhea (pellagra); poor metabolism of carbohydrates, amino acids and fatty acids.

Dosage range - RDA 13 mg. daily for females and 18 mg. daily for males; typical daily dosage range is 15-2000 mg. daily; therapeutic treatment dosage range is up to 6 grams daily. There are transient side effects to larger doses (above 75mg.) of niacin as it releases histamine. These include flushing, tingling, and possibly throbbing in the head. These last 20-30 min. Sustained release niacin should be taken with caution as it can be toxic to the liver.

Dietary sources - Best sources are organ meats, brewer's yeast, milk, legumes, and peanuts. Fish, poultry and lean meats are moderate sources.

Vitamin B6 (pyroxidine)

Function and Effect - B6 is required for the production of histamine, GABA, serotonin, norepinephrine, and acetylcholine; necessary in the growth of red blood cells and hemoglobin formation; required for glycogen to glucose conversion; metabolizes homocysteine, helping to prevent atherosclerosis; converts tryptophan to niacin and synthesizes it; reduces PMS symptoms in women who take oral contraceptives; helpful with depression; may be useful in preventing carpal tunnel syndrome.

Effects of depletion/deficiency - Neurological, circulatory, and dermatologic alterations; elevated homocysteine; PMS; lethargy; depression; sleep disturbances; anemia; nerve inflammation; dermatitis.

Dosage range - RDA 2 mg.; typical dosage range is 2-100 mg.; therapeutic doses are 10-100 mg. The U.S. Department of Agriculture cites that 80% of Americans
are deficient in this nutrient. Much of this nutrient is lost in cooking. Large doses of 2 grams or more a day have been found to be temporarily toxic to the neurological system.

Dietary sources - brewer's yeast, wheat germ, organ meat, legumes, bananas, potatoes.

Vitamin B12 (cobalamin)

Function and Effect - Assists in generating tetrahydrofolate in the synthesis of DNA; B12 enzymes are crucial for reducing RNA to DNA, playing a major role in replicating the genetic code; required for synthesis of the myelin sheath that surrounds nerves; helps red blood cells to mature; helps to metabolize carbohydrates, fats, proteins, methionine and folic acid.

Effects of depletion/deficiency -neurological changes; anemia; poor growth and repair of cells; fatigue; confusion, memory loss, and depression; loss of appetite; mouth and tongue changes; skin sensitivity; rashes (dermatitis);
peripheral neuropathy; poor blood clotting; sensitive to bruising. Chronic B12 deficiency causes the body to lose its ability to properly assimilate B12 from food. Injections are then necessary.

Dosage range -RDA 6 mcg.; typical dosage 100-2000 mcg. daily; not known to be toxic. Oral doses are poorly assimilated.

Dietary sources - organ meats, clams, oysters, beef, eggs, milk, chicken, cheese.

Note: Vegetarians who eat no dairy need to supplement B12.

Bifidobacteria Bifidum (bifudus)
Function and Effect - produces short chain fatty acids in the colon that discourages the growth of pathological bacteria, molds, and yeasts; fuels the cells that line the inner surface of the colon.

Effects of depletion/deficiency - chronic yeast infections; bloating and gas; constipation or diarrhea; bad breath

Dosage range - No RDA has been set. Typical preventive dosage range is 1-2 billion cfu. (colony forming units) daily; when taking antibiotics dosage range is 10-15 billion cfu. twice daily (combined with acidophilus). No toxicity is known.

Dietary sources - None. Must be obtained through probiotic supplements, kefir.

Biotin (Vitamin H, Vitamin Bw, Coenzyme R - considered a B vitamin)
Function and effect - metabolizes fats and carbohydrates to produce energy; waste removal from protein assimilation; proper oxygenation.

Effects of depletion/deficiency - depression, anorexia, cardiac problems, skin problems (dermatitis) that can also appear near nose and mouth, hair loss and loss of hair color, muscle aches, neuritis (tingling and numbness in hands and/or feet), splitting finger nails.

Dosage range - RDA 0.3 mg; typical doses 30+ mcg. daily; therapeutic doses up to 3 mg. daily. No toxicity.

Dietary sources - found in most plant and animal foods (brewer's yeast, liver, and bananas are some best sources), and synthesized in 'good' bacteria of intestines.

Note: Biotin deficiency is thought to be rare. This statement is theoretical only. It does not take into consideration diets consisting of denatured foods or drugs taken that interfere with the assimilation of biotin.

Vitamin C (ascorbic acid)

Function and Effect - Concentrated in many tissues but most abundant in adrenal glands; obtained entirely through diet; synthesizes collagen and elastin (the most abundant protein in the body); antioxidant; hormonal response; increases HDL cholesterol; decreases LDL cholesterol; decreases lipoproteins (implicated
in atherosclerosis); dissolves atherosclerotic plaque; increases protective white blood cells; increases interferon production; increases infection fighting antibodies (IgA, IgG, IgM); modulates prostaglandin synthesis; prevents cervical dysplasia; reduces bronchial spasms in those with respiratory diseases; detoxifies heavy metals; promotes healing of wounds and broken bones.

Dosage range - RDA 60 mg. daily; typical dosage 60-12,000 mg. daily in divided doses; therapeutic doses 500 mg. - 20 grams. Non-toxic; side effect from higher doses can be diarrhea, some gas, bloating. Vit C supplements with mineral ascorbates

do not usually cause this problem. Vitamin C produces high amounts of
oxalic acid. Those with compromised kidneys or a history of gout should consult a professional prior to using more than 500 mg. daily.

Dietary sources - fresh fruits and vegetables.

Calcium

Function and Effect - Most abundant mineral in the body, 99% of which is in bones and teeth (1% in body fluids and cells); regulates heart beat; assists in protein metabolism and fat digestion; initiates contraction of muscles; assists in maintaining normal blood pressure; prevents osteoporosis.

Effects of depletion/deficiency - Bone deformity (rickets); tooth decay; nervous disorders; insomnia; hypertension; soft or brittle bones; heart palpitations; muscle cramps.

Dosage range - RDA depends on age.

0-6 months 400 mg.

6-12 months 600 mg.

1-5 years 800 mg.

6-10 " 800-1200 mg.

11-24 " 1200 mg.

25-65 males 1000 mg.

25-50 females 1000 mg.

Pregnancy 1200-1500 mg.

51-65 females taking estrogen 1000 mg.

51-65 " no estrogen 1500 mg.

over 65 1500 mg.

Typical dosage 800-2000 mg. (therapeutic doses same). Not usually toxic; may possibly interfere with absorption of magnesium, iron, and zinc.

Dietary sources - Dark green leafy vegetables, broccoli, whole grains, legumes, nuts, milk, dairy products.

Notes: Excess phosphorus (soft drinks, animal proteins) increases calcium excretion via urine, causing the body to leach calcium from the bones. Cow's milk may not be a good source of calcium or any other nutrient for the following reasons: many people are lactose intolerant; the foreign proteins in cow's milk frequently cause food allergies; cow's milk contains an enzyme that can cause damage to arteries; antibodies to a particular bovine oxidase appears
in the blood of people with atherosclerosis.

CoQ10 (Coenzyme Q10, ubiquinone)

Function and Effect - Most of the CoQ10 we require is made by our cells in a 17-step process that requires several vitamins and numerous trace minerals.Deficiencies or depletions of any of these vitamins and minerals will interfere
in our ability to manufacture CoQ10. CoQ10 produces energy in the mitochondria of every cell, and is particularly abundant in the mitochondria of the heart. It is a coenzyme for a number of other enzymes that are involved in producing ATP, a high energy fuel for all cells. Protects against free radical damage; protects against toxic side effects of beta blocker, antibiotic, and psychiatric drugs;
helpful in periodontal disease.

Effects of depletion/deficiency - weakening of the immune system; lack of energy; cardiomyopathy; mitral valve prolapse;

cardiac arrhythmias; congestive heart failure; angina; hypertension; gingivitis. The cardiovascular system and the heart is the first to be affected by deficient/depleted CoQ10.

Dosage range - No RDA set; Typical dosage range 30-100 mg. daily; those who are taking any prescription drugs that deplete CoQ10, or have heart disease should supplement with CoQ10 in the 200-300 mg. a day range. Higher doses are possible if advised by a professional. There are no known toxicities or side effects.

Dietary sources - Although Coenzyme Q compounds exist in all plants and animals, it is believed that we cannot get enough for supplementing purposes from dietary sources.

Note: Many of the drugs given to people to allegedly arrest or prevent heart disease deplete CoQ10 by interfering in its production. This leads to further damage to the heart and circulatory system. The statin drugs, used for reducing cholesterol, severely deplete CoQ10. The description of rhabdomyolosis, a possible side effect of statin drugs, is consistent with the symptoms of severeCoQ10 depletion.

Vitamin D (calciferol)

Function and Effect - Vitamin D is a hormone precursor that is made by the body when exposed to sunlight. Without adequate sunshine, Vitamin D deficiency occurs. Vitamin D is produced in the kidneys and converted into very potent analogs of Vitamin D in the liver. It plays a vital role in the mineralization and demineralization of bones; regulates levels and promotes absorption of calcium and phosphorus; believed to help in the prevention of osteoporosis (the parathyroid gland becomes stimulated when calcium levels are low, and leaches calcium from bones); inhibits lymphoma, leukemia, breast and colon cancer cells; stimulates lymph circulation by boosting macrophage activity (macrophages clean up toxins in lymph fluids); can be helpful in the form of direct sunlight for those with psoriasis.

Effects of depletion/deficiency - rickets (in children); bone weakness; osteoporosis; osteomalacia; rheumatic pains; muscle weakness; tooth decay; increased incidence of pelvis and hip fractures; gradual loss of hearing.

Dosage range - RDA 400 IU (International Units) daily; therapeutic dosages 1000-5,000 IU daily. An overabundance of Vitamin D (highly unusual and reversible) can cause calcium deposits in arteries, lungs, kidneys, heart, and ears. Symptoms of toxicity include constipation, headache, nausea, vomiting, weakness, shortness of breath, dull ache in kidney area.

Dietary sources - small amounts in liver, cream, butter, egg yolks. Found most regularly in milk, which is fortified with Vitamin. Most people in the Western World are deficient.

Vitamin E (alpha tocopherol)

Function and Effect - Most important fat-soluble antioxidant: Prevents free radical damage by insuring the integrity and stability of membranes and cellulartissues; protects blood vessels; antioxidant properties protect eyes; protects LDL cholesterol against oxidation; protects against free radical damage during exercise.

Effects of depletion/deficiency - bruising; dry skin; dry hair;

eczema; psoriasis; poor wound healing; anemia; PMS; hot flashes; cataracts; fibrocystic tumors in breasts; sterility; muscle weakness; liver, pancreatic, colon, rectal, cervical, oral, lung cancers.

Dosage range - RDA 30 IU (international units) daily; typical dosage 100-1200 IU daily. Toxicity is rarely reported, but can occur for a minority of people when taking over 1,000 IU daily. Symptoms of toxicity are: double vision, fatigue, muscle weakness, nausea, headache, gastric distress.

Dietary sources - Vitamin E is widely available in foods. Extra-virgin olive oil; seeds; nuts; whole grains; leafy greens; avocadoes; asparagus; Brussels sprouts; spinach.

Note - Dry Vitamin E supplements in the form of d-alpha tocopherol are more bioavailable than dl-alpha tocopherol, which is synthetic Vitamin E. Those taking anti-coagulant drugs should use Vitamin E with caution.

Folic Acid (folacin)

Function and Effect - Folic acid is a common vitamin deficiency. Synthesizes DNA and RNA; needed to convert homocysteine to methionine; prevents some birth defects, including cleft lip, cleft palate and spina bifida; necessary for healthy blood cells; supplementing with folic acid prevents and reverses
cervical dysplasia.

Effects of depletion/deficiency - damages DNA metabolism in cells of vagina and cervix, stomach and intestines; more frequent infections; nausea; anorexia; headache; fatigue; hair loss; elevated homocysteine levels; cervical dysplasia;

megaloblastic anemia; birth defects.

Dosage range - RDA 200 mcg daily; typical dosage range 200-800 mcg daily; therapeutic dosage range 5,000-10,000 mcg daily. Folic acid is not toxic, but can mask a deficiency of Vitamin B12. This can be avoided by limiting dosage to 800 mcg or less.

Dietary sources - Folic acid is readily available, and can be found in liver, eggs, brewer's yeast, cabbage, cauliflower, dark green leafy vegetables, broccoli, Brussels sprouts, beets, cantaloupe, orange juice, lima and kidney beans, wheat germ, whole grains.

Notes - Women who are pregnant and lactating need higher doses than the RDA of folic acid. Further, before choosing to become pregnant, all women should be tested for their folic acid status. As the use of oral contraceptives has increased over the years, so has the number of women diagnosed as having cervical dysplasia. Oral contraceptives severely deplete folic acid, and all women taking these drugs should supplement with folic acid. Those with a history
of colon cancer and ulcerative colitis can benefit from taking folic acid supplements.

Glutathione

Function and Effect - performs antioxidant activity in red blood cells and mitochondria; synthesizes fatty acids; one of a group of nutrients that supports hepatic (liver) detoxification of alcohol, cigarette smoke and large amounts of acetaminophen and aspirin; reduces free radical damage from radiation; crucial to the development and function of lymphocytes, macrophages and other types of immune cells.

Effects of depletion/deficiency - increased free radical damage; compromised immune system function; poor hepatic detoxification; hair loss.

Dosage range - RDA not established; typical dosage 500-3,000 mg daily in divided doses. There are no known side effects or toxicity.

Dietary sources - raw vegetables; fresh fruit; meat; fish; avocado; walnuts; asparagus.

Note - When purchasing this supplement, be sure it is in its reduced form. Unreduced glutathione is not active.

Inositol

Function and Effect - part of the phospholipids and the B complex vitamins (phospholipids are like tri-glycerides except that the first hydroxyl of the glycerine molecule has a polar phosphate containing group in place of the fatty acid) which help cells respond appropriately to external stimuli. It also helps with the production of an omega-6 fatty acid PUFA called arachidonic acid which

is necessary to cell membrane function. When PGE-1 is lacking, arachidonic acid leaks from cell membranes and fuels the production of the inflammatory series-2 prostaglandins (PGE-2). PGE-2 also promotes platelet aggregation and causes the kidneys to retain sodium.

There are three forms of inositol that are not well understood. Studies are currently underway. Promise is shown in the area of addictions, the " mental illnesses " , and chronic fatigue syndrome.

Effects of depletion - improper cell function. Depletion rarely happens if one eats grains, nuts or organ meats.

Dosage range - No RDA. Typical dosage is 100-1000 mg. daily.

Dietary sources - grains, nuts, beans, organ and muscle meats.- Insitol depletion (most likely to happen if diagnosed with chronic fatigue syndrome).

Iron

Function and Effect - Iron binds oxygen to hemoglobin and transports, as necessary, to all tissues in the body. Iron also plays a role in the synthesis of dopamine and serotonin transmitters. Healthy immune response is dependent upon iron. Iron also assists liver detoxification enzymes. Iron assists the amino acid, carnitine, which is necessary to fatty acid metabolism. Collagen and elastin are dependent upon iron.

Effects of depletion - fatigue, compromised immune function, anemia, hair loss, brittle nails and other nail problems, headache, difficulty breathing when performing physical tasks or activities.

Dosage range - RDA 15 mg. females; 10 mg. males. Typical dosage is 10-50 mg. daily. Toxic doses of iron are rare as the body will not store an overabundance of it. Iron overdose can happen to people who are addicted to alcohol. Due to liver damage, iron can be absorbed in excess. There is also a genetic defect that allows the body to absorb too much iron.

Dietary sources - liver, poultry, fish, other organ meats, vegetables, dried beans, and small amounts in grains.

Lactobacillus Acidophilus

Function and Effect - Lactobacillus acidophilus inhabits the small intestine as beneficial bacteria. This bacteria is easily destroyed by antibiotics. Produces Vitamin K and numerous B vitamins in the intestinal tract; produces natural antibiotics in the GI tract that help to prevent infection; creates enzymes that assist in digesting proteins, fats and dairy products; metabolizes cholesterol.

Effect of depletion/deficiency - chronic vaginal yeast infections; bloating; gas; constipation or diarrhea; halitosis (bad breath).

Dosage range - No RDA established. See BIFIDOBACTERIA BIFIDUM DOSAGE RANGE for dosage suggestions. There are no side effects or toxicities.

Dietary sources - yogurt; acidophilus milk (see CALCIUM NOTES for concerns about milk).

Vitamin K (phytonadione)

Function and Effect - necessary for the production of several blood clotting factors; helps to synthesize a protein unique to the bones which assists in drawing calcium to bone tissue. Vitamin K is actually three vitamins called the quinones.

Effect of depletion/deficiency - osteoporosis; osteomalacia; hemorrhage. Newborn infants are more likely to have a Vitamin K deficiency than adults.

Dosage range - RDA 60 mcg women; 80 mcg men. Typical dosage 30-100 mcg.

Therapeutic doses can be higher, but because large doses of Vitamin K can be toxic a prescription is necessary. Infants can develop a fatal form of jaundice from too much Vitamin K.

Dietary sources - any type of cabbage; green leafy vegetables; liver. Vitamin K is synthesized by intestinal bacteria; therefore, we needn't get most of our Vitamin K from food.

Notes - In order for the small intestine to absorb Vitamin K, the appropriate amounts of bile and pancreatic juices are necessary. If an adult were to present with the rare deficiency of Vitamin K, I would first recommend digestive enzymes. It is far more common for people to lack appropriate amounts of digestive enzymes than Vitamin K.

*If taking Warfarin (Coumadin) do NOT supplement with vitamin k, as it blocks the blood thinning action of the medication.

Magnesium

Function and Effect - cofactor in the production of ATP; necessary for synthesis of DNA and RNA; involved in hundreds of enzymatic reactions; metabolizes proteins, carbohydrates and fats; crucial to muscle and nerve tissues; prevents tooth decay by binding calcium to tooth enamel; helps to metabolize calcium and synthesize Vitamin D; relaxes blood vessels; acts as an anticoagulant; blocks calcium uptake; reduces risk of cardiovascular disease; increases oxygen to heart tissues.

Effect of depletion/deficiency - Mild deficiency is commonplace in the US. Symptoms are depression, confusion, anxiety, fear, irritability, fatigue, muscle cramps, weakness, insomnia, loss of appetite, kidney stones, osteoporosis, gastric disorders. Processed foods contribute to the magnesium deficiencies in

Americans. Most fertilizers used by commercial farmers do not contain magnesium. When food is refined, it loses up to 85% of its natural magnesium. Magnesium deficiency can cause cardiac arrest. Death following cardiac episodes is more likely to occur in people who are deficient in magnesium. Magnesium deficiency is also noted in those who abuse alcohol, have diabetes, liver disease and/or kidney disease.

Dosage range - RDA 400 mg daily; typical dosage 400-1,000 mg daily; therapeutic dose 500-1500 mg daily. Toxicity is rare.

Dietary sources - green leafy vegetables; whole grains; nuts; legumes.

Notes - When I.V. magnesium is given when a heart attack begins, a 70% decrease in deaths is realized. Supplementing magnesium would be helpful to most, if not all, people.

Phosphorous

Function and Effect - Phosphorous is the second most abundant mineral in the body and is involved in every metabolic process. Assists in the transportation of lipids across cellular membranes and through the body; necessary to the integrity of teeth and bones; crucial to protein synthesis and cellular reproduction; a partner of many coenzymes.

Effects of depletion/deficiency - Phosphorous deficiency is rare. The effects of depletion are numerous and beyond the scope of this guide. People with celiacdisease, Crohn's disease, malabsorption syndromes, alcohol addictions and kidney malfunction are most prone to phosphorous depletion.

Dosage range - RDA 800-1,200 mg daily.

Dietary sources - Studies say that most Americans consume too much phosphorous. An abundance of phosphorous is found in animal protein and cola soft drinks.

Notes - Too much phosphorous can inhibit calcium absorption and contribute to hyperthyroidism, calcium deposits in soft tissues and decreases in bone mass. Regular use of antacids that contain aluminum can deplete phosphorous.

Potassium

Function and Effect - Potassium is one of three major electrolytes and is the primary electrolyte at work inside our cells. Crucial to muscle contraction, heartbeat, nerve conduction, maintaining balance of water throughout body; helps to prevent hypertension; can reduce blood pressure.

Effects of depletion/deficiency - muscle weakness; fatigue; cardiac arrhythmia; constipation; poor reflexes; dizziness; nervous disorders. Potassium can also be depleted by chronic stress, kidney failure, malnutrition, acidosis (diabetic), alcohol abuse, caffeine, excessive sugar or salt.

Dosage range - no RDA established; typical dose if needed is 60-99 mg. Potassium toxicity occurs mostly from malfunctioning adrenal glands and/or kidney failure. Symptoms of this are difficulty breathing, diminished cardiac activity, confusion, and/or numbness in extremities.

Dietary sources - fresh vegetables, fruits, meat, milk (see NOTES under CALCIUM).

Sodium

Function and Effect - As one of three major electrolytes in the body, sodium is the primary extracellular electrolyte in body fluids. Sodium helps to regulate blood pressure, the balance of alkaline/acid in the lymph and blood, and the transport and excretion of carbon dioxide. It assists in making the cell walls permeable and plays a vital role in muscle contraction and nerve function.

Effects of depletion/deficiency - Only a few conditions can cause sodium deficiency. They are excessive perspiration and the absence of water, severe diarrhea, starvation, vomiting. Deficiency symptoms can include poor concentration, muscle weakness, dehydration, loss of appetite, memory loss.

Dosage range - No RDA established; 1-3 grams per day will suffice. Most people consume up to 30 times more sodium daily than needed. Toxic effects can be edema and increased blood pressure.

Dietary sources - Sodium is found in meats, grains and vegetables. Negligible amounts can be found in fruits.

Notes - Common table salt is a concentrated form of sodium. It has many additives and the ratio of potassium to sodium is not compatible with the body. Processed foods contain very high amounts of sodium and contain no potassium,
making them even worse for the body than common table salt. Solar-dried or Celtic sea salt is a healthy replacement for table salt.

Selenium

Function and Effect - Selenium functions as an antioxidant that can prevent cardiovascular disease and cancer (low selenium levels are correlated with high rates of cancer). Destroys mercury and cadmium; increases NK (natural killer) cell activity, antiviral activity and T lymphocytes; helps to convert T4 thyroid

hormone to T3; is a potent anti-inflammatory; boosts Vitamin E antioxidant
actions.

Effects of depletion/deficiency - undesirable changes to the pancreas and heart; compromised immune system; sore muscles; weakness of red blood cells; increased incidence of many cancers; cardiomyopathy.

Dosage range - RDA 55 mcg daily women; 70 mcg daily men. **Typical dosage 50-200 mcg daily**. Therapeutic dosage 50-500 mcg daily. Higher doses have been used. Selenium can be toxic. Symptoms are breath that smells like garlic, skin lesions, hair and nail loss, malfunction of the nervous system, digestive problems.

Dietary sources - whole grains, cucumbers, cabbage, radishes, celery, eggs, liver, seafood, garlic,.

Note - The selenium content of foods is related to the selenium content of soil. It is common today for our farm soils to have less selenium. Convenience foods lack adequate selenium.

Tyrosine

Function and Effect - necessary for the production of thyroid hormones; facilitates synthesis of norepinephrine, epinephrine, dopamine.

Effects of depletion/deficiency - metabolic disturbances; hypothyroidism; depression and emotional disturbances.

Dosage range - no RDA established; dosage range 1,000-5,000 mg daily. No known toxicities. Can cause some symptoms at very high doses.

Dietary sources - poultry, meats, wheat, corn, eggs, milk (see

NOTES under CALCIUM).

Notes - Tyrosine supplements are effective for some people suffering from depression.

Zinc

Function and Effect - protects DNA from damage; participates in cellular division, protein synthesis, gene expression, DNA and RNA synthesis; helps to digest proteins; involved in numerous activities of the immune system and hundreds of enzymes; controls the release of Vitamin A from the liver; crucial to ovulation, fertilization, sperm maturation; regulator of sensory perceptions; assists in conversion of thyroid hormones T4 to T3; possesses anti inflammatory properties; keeps prostate gland healthy and prevents benign hyperplasia.

Effects of depletion/deficiency - Zinc deficiencies, though mild, are common in the US. This is due to zinc-depleted soils, processed foods, convenience foods and low-protein/low-calorie diets. Alcohol can also deplete zinc. Symptoms include impaired sense of taste and smell, night blindness, nystagmus, slow healing of wounds, infections, depression, acne, menstrual problems. Zinc depletion is also seen in liver and kidney diseases, celiac disease, IBD (inflammatory bowel diseases), macular degeneration and diabetes.

Dosage range - RDA 12 mg daily women; 15 mg daily men. Therapeutic dosage 10-15mg daily. Not toxic below 150 mg daily.

Dietary sources - seafood, liver, lean meats, whole grains, eggs.

Notes - Low animal protein and grains high in phytates can cause children to fail to mature sexually and show signs of dwarfism and hypogonadism. Pregnant women need more zinc than the RDA. Deficiency in this can cause birth defects.

Chapter 7: Food Lists for Autoimmunity

"He that takes medicine and neglects diet wastes the skills of the physician." ~ Chinese proverb

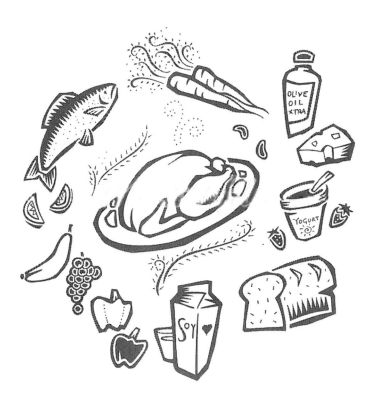

The Following foods are safe and healthy for those affected by autoimmune disorders:

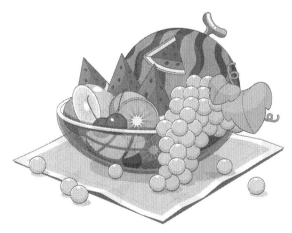

- Acai
- Adzuki Beans
- Almonds
- Anchovies**
- Apple Cider Vinegar
- Apples
- Apricots
- Asparagus
- Arugula
- Artichokes
- Avocado
- Bananas (In Moderation)
- Basil
- Beets
- Bison
- Black Beans
- Blackberries
- Blueberries
- Bok Choy
- Borage Oil
- Brazil Nuts
- Broccoli
- Brown Rice
- Brussell Sprouts
- Cabbage
- Cantalope
- Carrots
- Cashews
- Cauliflower
- Cayenne Pepper
- Celery
- Chia Seeds
- Cherries
- Chicken (Lean, White Meat)
- Cilantro
- Cinnamon
- Cloves
- Cocoa
- Coconut Oil
- Cod
- Cranberries
- Cucumber
- Cumin
- Edamame
- Eggs (Cage Free)
- Eggplant
- Endive
- Fennel
- Figs
- Flax seed
- Garbanzo Beans
- Ginger
- Goat's Milk
- Goji Berries
- Grapeseed Oil
- Green Beans
- Haddock**
- Hazelnuts
- Hemp seeds
- Kale
- Kefir
- Kiwi Fruit
- Leeks
- Lemons
- Lentils
- Licorice
- Limes
- Mackerel (North Atlantic)**
- Mango
- Mint
- Mushrooms
- Mustard Greens
- Navy Beans
- Nutmeg
- Oatmeal (Not Instant)
- Olive Oil (Extra Virgin)
- Oranges (In Moderation)
- Oregano
- Papaya
- Parsnips
- Peaches
- Pears
- Peas
- Pecans
- Pineapple-- Fresh
- Pine Nuts
- Pinto Beans
- Pumpkin
- Quinoa
- Radishes
- Raspberries
- Romaine
- Rosemary
- Rhubarb
- Rutabaga
- Salmon (Wild Caught)**
- Sardines**
- Sea Vegetables
- Soy Nuts*
- Spinach
- Squash
- Strawberries
- Sweet Potato
- Swiss Chard

- Tarragon
- Thyme
- Soy Products (Tofu, Tempeh, Etc)*
- Trout

- Tuna
- Turkey (White Meat)
- Turnips
- Walnuts
- Watercress

- Wheat Grass
- White Beans
- Yogurt (unsweetened)
- Venison
- Zucchini

** Wild-Caught Only—Not Farm Raised

*In Moderation

Foods to Avoid In Autoimmunity

- Alfalfa seeds and sprouts-- should be avoided because they contain an amino acid called L-canavanine. This amino acid can aggravate the symptoms of lupus and other autoimmune disorders
- Artificial Sweeteners, Including Aspartame, Saccharin, Splenda
- Chemical Preservatives, Coloring, Flavors
- Corn
- Cured Meats (Lunchmeat, Ham, Etc)
- Dairy
- Gluten
- Herbs- such as andrographis, echinacea, eleutherococcus, garlic, ginseng, and Panax – These stimulate the immune system, and could lead to a flare.
- High Fructose Corn Syrup
- High Protein Foods (especially important if you have kidney disease)

- Nightshade Vegetables (Peppers, Tomatoes, White Potatoes)
- Oils--like corn, poppy seed, safflower, and sunflower encourage autoimmune flare episodes
- Peanuts
- Processed/Packaged Foods
- Red Meat
- Refined Foods, such as white breads, pastas, and sugar
- Soda Pop, Energy Drinks, Alcohol
- Trans Fats, Saturated Fats
- Wheat

Chapter 8: Oral Disease In Lupus and Autoimmune Disorders

"If you don't take care of your body, where are you going to live?"
~Unknown

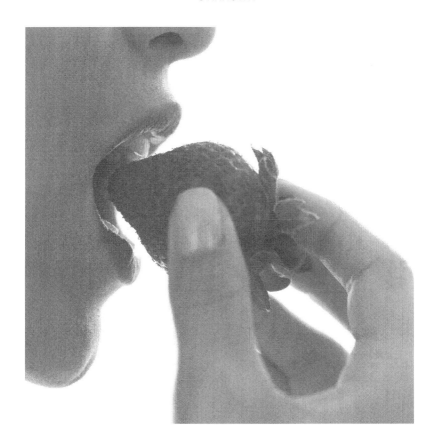

The oral mucosae,or lining of the mouth, is one of the most common targets in lupus erythematosus (LE) and autoimmune disease patients. Oral mucosal disorders certainly affect nutrition—with pain in the mouth, decreasing the ability to eat a variety of foods.

Next, is the western medical treatment of oral lesions in autoimmunity, followed by specific measures you can take yourself, for these conditions.

Autoimmune Mouth Issues

Oral Apthae (canker sores)

In the medical literature, oral apthae often are referred to as recurrent apthous stomatitis. These sores, or lesions, affect up to 15 percent of the normal population.

Conditions associated with a higher frequency of oral apthae are:

- systemic lupus erythematosus (SLE)
- inflammatory bowel disease (IBD)
- celiac disease
- acquired immune deficiency syndrome (AIDS) and other causes of immunodeficiency states
- Behcet's Disease, a rare disease characterized by oral, genital, and skin ulcers as well as eye inflammation and systemic vasculitis.

Description: The oral apthae lesions are often small (less than 1 cm), painful, and have a tendency to occur on the buccal mucosae (inner cheeks) of the mouth. The lesions tend to last up to two to three weeks. The main mimicker of apthae is herpes (a.k.a. fever blisters). In herpes, the ulcers often affect the lips and gums. They tend to appear in groups and to be preceded by fluid-filled blisters.

Oral apthae in LE patients tend to last longer, be larger, and appear most often on the hard palate, or roof of the mouth. The most important feature of apthae in LE patients is the strong association of these oral ulcers with an internal organ flare of the systemic lupus disease.

Treatments: The most effective treatment for LE apthae overall, is to control the SLE with immunosuppressive therapy. This usually is based on the combination of systemic corticosteroids with anti-metabolites, such as azathioprine (Imuran) or mycophenolate mofetil (CellCept) with cyclophosphamide. In addition, folic acid (1 gram daily) has been proven helpful in many cases.

Additional treatment may consist of high-potency corticosteroids placed directly upon the lesion, such as kenalog in orabase, clobetasol gel (4-5 times a day); or medicines taken by mouth, such as prednisone. In addition, Magic Mouthwash—see below, can help speed healing and provide comfort.

Mucosal discoid lupus erythematosus:

Discoid lupus erythematosus (DLE) is the most common form of chronic cutaneous lupus erythematosus. The head and neck are most commonly affected areas. Very few people with DLE have associated systemic LE.

However, certain subsets of people DLE have a stronger relationship to systemic lupus. These are people with:

- disseminated DLE (DLE lesions above and below the neck);
- palmoplantar DLE (DLE lesion on the palms of the hands and soles of the feet);
- familial DLE or familial SLE (first-degree relatives with DLE or SLE);
- mucosal DLE (DLE lesions affecting mouth and rarely, other mucous membranes).

Description: DLE of the oral mucosa occurs only in the setting of cutaneous DLE. The most commonly affected location is the inner cheeks, and often there will be associated lip lesions. Usually these will be asymptomatic (presenting no symptoms), but when ulcerated they become quite painful.

The lesions resemble red plaques surrounded by lacy whitish areas. Mucosal DLE lesions are much like lesions seen in a very common disease called lichen planus. The presence of DLE-associated lesions on the skin and lips should prompt to the exclusion of oral DLE in patients with "lichen planus-like" mouth lesions.

Treatments: Treatment of mucosal DLE are be based on a combination of topical and systemic therapy. Topical therapy consists of high potency corticosteroids (clobetasol gel 4-5 times a day). Hydroxychloroquine (Plaquenil) 200 mg twice daily, is often highly effective for oral DLE. Rarely, severe cases may require systemic immunosuppressive drugs such as azathioprine. mycophenolate mofetil, or leflunomide (Arava).

Oral Candidiasis

Candida albicans is the most frequent cause of fungal human disease in general, and is the most common cause of oral fungal involvement. The organism is a normal inhabitant of the oral cavity in 30 to 40% of the population. When the bacterial flora of the oral cavity is disturbed by antibiotic therapy, or in individuals who have diabetes mellitus, xerostomia (dry-mouth), weakened immunity, immunosuppression from medications for autoimmune illness, or severe debilitation, this otherwise harmless microorganism multiplies to cause overt lesions.

Oral Candidiasis takes the form of a superficial, curdy, gray to white membrane that can be readily scraped off to reveal an underlying red, inflammatory base. In the milder expressions, there is minimal ulceration of the mucosal surface, which does not penetrate deeper into the tissues. More severe oral infections may produce mucosal ulceration and a correspondingly greater inflammatory reaction.

Oral yeast infections may cause a burning sensation, tenderness, or sometimes pain around the affected area of the mouth—most commonly the tongue and throat. Spicy and salty foods will cause discomfort because of the increased sensitivity of the affected area.

Treatment: The underlying systemic conditions (such as diabetes, malnutrition, and anemia) and the discontinuation of broad-spectrum antibiotics are recommended for the first approaches. Local resistance can be improved by good oral hygiene and by leaving dentures out as much as possible.

The five drugs that are used for antifungal therapy are gentian violet, nystatin, miconazole, clotrimazole, and ketoconazole. Nystatin has been the standard drug used for oral candidal infections for the last 35 years. Each of these drugs is absorbed poorly from the gastrointestinal tract but is excellent for topical use on mucous membrane and skin lesions. Most dentists and physicians stress the importance of continuing antifungal therapy at least 2 weeks following disappearance of signs and symptoms of oral lesions.

Ok, so that was rather depressing! What can you do, on your own, to treat and prevent these problems?

Remedies For Sore Mouth/Ulcers

- Drink Plenty of Water—Unless Kidney Disease!
- Salt water rinses
- Aloe Vera Gel-dab on spot
- Clove or Oregano oil-dab on spot
- Zinc lozenges (5mg)-1 four times daily

- Vitamin C (500mg)-1 four times daily
- L-Lysine- 1,000 mg L-lysine three times daily with meals, while sore is present, then 500mg three times daily for one week, following healing
- Hydrogen Peroxide- Rinse twice daily
- Periogard Mouthwash (Chlorhexadine gluconate)= 10 ml swish twice daily

As someone who suffers from Lupus, and frequent oral ulcers—these do work, but please--Be in touch with your doctor—if the ulcers do not improve rapidly—make an appointment!

Magic Mouthwash—Excellent for Sore Mouth!
Best Prescription Recipe
2 ounces each of:
Maalox--Coats
Benadryl (Diphenhydramine) Elixir 12.5mg/5ml (Childrens)--Anti-inflammatory
Nystatin Suspension
Prednisolone Syrup 15mg/5ml
Lidocaine Viscous-numbs
Swish and spit or swallow 10ml every 4 hours as needed. Also can dab with a Q Tip on Individual Sores.

Best Non-Prescription
2 ounces each of:
Maalox

Benadryl (Diphenhydramine) Elixir 12.5mg/5ml (Childrens)

Can Add 5 Drops Clove, Tea Tree or Oregano Oil, or Anbesol 2 droppers—Numbing.

Essential Supplements for Oral Health

B-Complex 50mg—1 Daily

Acidophilius-- 3 billion cultures daily

Zinc—50 mg daily

Vitamin C—1000-2000 mg daily

L-Lysine—500mg daily--maintenence

References:

Burgess, JA, Johnson, BD, Sommers, E. Pharmacological management of recurrent oral mucosal ulceration. *Drugs.* 1990;39(1):54–65.

Strohecker J, ed. Alternative medicine: the definitive guide. Fife, Wash.: Future Medicine, 1995:264.

Chapter 9 : Essential Supplements in Autoimmunity

"The best and most efficient pharmacy is within your own system." ~Robert C. Peale

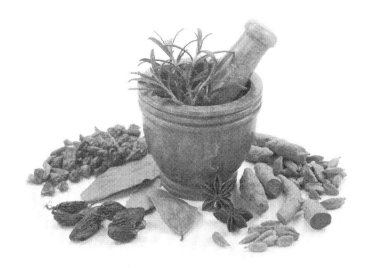

Omega 3 Fatty Acids

The essential fatty acids in fish oil, flaxseed oil,and evening primrose oil (or borage oil) act as natural anti-inflammatories, protecting your joints, kidneys, and skin. Fish Oil

Fish oil contains omega-3 fatty acids, an essential fatty acid that supports heart health by reducing the risk of conditions like coronary artery disease.

According to the Lupus Foundation of America (LFA) women with lupus have a 5 to 10 times higher risk for heart disease, so fish oil could be important in maintaining good health. Research is also being done to confirm the anti-inflammatory properties of omega-3 fatty acids, which could benefit lupus.

Two clinical studies found that taking fish oil reduced lupus severity (Duffy, 2004; Walton, 1991). Another study found that taking fish oil reduced the level of serum lipids in people with lupus (Clark, 1993), which may be useful as they are at a greater risk of developing heart disease.

Flax Seed Oil

Flaxseed and flaxseed oil contain a type of omega-3 fatty acid called alpha-linolenic acid (ALA). The UMMC says ALA benefits arthritis and decreases inflammation. ALA may also improve kidney function affected by lupus.

Evening primrose oil, black currant, or borage oil contain the essential fatty acid GLA, which reduces joint inflammation. Take up to 2.8 grams of GLA daily.

Vitamins and Minerals (From Whole Food Vitamins)

A researcher from the University of Hawaii published a review article in 2000 in the "Journal of Renal Nutrition" about nutrition and lupus. Vitamin E, vitamin A, selenium, and calcium with vitamin D were all listed as possible beneficial compounds for lupus. Selenium is an antioxidant that supports immune function and according to the UMMC, people with arthritis, another condition affected by inflammation, are often selenium deficient. Vitamin E is also an antioxidant and preliminary research shows that when used with traditional medications, it may decrease the pain associated with arthritis. Researchers at the Medical University of South Carolina conducted a literature review and concluded in a 2008 article in "Current Opinion in Rheumatology," that lupus patients are often vitamin D deficient and supplementation could be beneficial.

Vitamin D

Vitamin D is an essential nutrient, and the precursor to the active form is produced in the skin after absorbing ultra-violet light. Other sources of vitamin D include fatty fish like salmon and mackerel; fortified foods like margarine, milk, and breakfast cereals; and vitamin D supplements (Berdanier, 2008).

Studies have shown that vitamin D may be important in reducing the risk of lupus (Cantorna, 2004). It has been shown that higher blood levels of vitamin d are associated with less severe lupus disease activity (Amital, 2010).

Vitamin D is another fat-soluble immune system powerhouse. Also known as the sunshine vitamin, most people can get the recommended daily allowance by going outside on a sunny day with fully exposed skin -- say, wearing a bathing suit -- for up to 15 minutes. Muscles rely on vitamin D for proper functioning, and nerves need the nutrient for transporting messages from around the body to the brain. Results of a study that looked at people with lupus were published by the journal "Current Opinion in Rheumatology" in September 2008. The study found that vitamin D reverses immune irregularities consistent with lupus. In a July 2011 article, the "New York Daily News" reported that the Feinstein Institute for Medical Research has begun studying the effects of vitamin D supplementation on lupus patients in the hope that the vitamin reduces disease flares.

Two observational studies found that women with systemic lupus erythematosus have significantly lower levels of 25-hydroxy vitamin D (Toloza, 2010; Borba, 2009). Another study found that, while 22% of healthy control women had a deficiency in vitamin D, 69% of women with lupus exhibited a deficiency in this vitamin (Ritterhouse, 2011).

Reduced levels of vitamin D in people with lupus may be due to one or both of two possible scenarios:

1. The deficiency is related to the disease itself; or
2. The deficiency is caused/exacerbated by avoiding sun exposure due to increased photosensitivity of individuals with lupus.

As discussed above, lupus and some of its treatments can cause bone loss and lead to osteoporosis. Healthy levels of vitamin D are necessary to help the body absorb calcium and keep bones as strong as possible and this is especially important in individuals with lupus.

Doseage: 2,000-8,000 IU daily vitamin D3, depending upon 25-hydroxy vitamin D levels, which should be 50-80 ng/ml for optimal health. Consult with your physician.

Individuals consuming more than 2000 IU/day of vitamin D (from diet and supplements) should periodically obtain a serum 25-hydroxy vitamin D measurement.

Do not exceed 10000 IU per day unless recommended by your doctor.

Vitamin D supplementation is not recommended for individuals with hypercalcemia (high blood calcium levels).

People with kidney disease, certain medical conditions (such as hyperparathyroidism or sarcoidosis), and those who use cardiac glycosides (digoxin) or thiazide diurectics should consult a physician before using supplemental vitamin D.

Bromelain

Pineapples are high in the enzyme bromelain, which may reduce inflammation and relieve pain, stiffness, redness and swelling in the joints of those suffering from lupus or RA, according to the University of Maryland Medical Center. Bromelain not only helps reduce inflammation but also aids the body in the digestion of protein. Bromelain supplements are as helpful as eating fresh pineapple and may be made even more effective by consuming them with turmeric supplements, which also reduces inflammation. If you take them as supplements, consume the bromelain between meals rather than with meals for the best results to reduce inflammation. If you prefer to eat pineapple, choose only fresh fruits and eat the fruit or juice it to obtain the most bromelain. Both bromelain and turmeric can thin the blood, so speak to your health provider if you take blood-thinning medicines before starting these treatments.

Bromelain is very safe to use on an ongoing basis. You might consider bromelain whenever your doctor recommends that you try using a nonsteroidal anti-inflammatory drug (NSAID), such as aspirin or ibuprofen.

Bromelain is not actually a single substance, but rather a collection of protein-digesting enzymes (also called proteolytic enzymes) found in pineapple juice and in the stem of pineapple plants.

Bromelain is definitely useful as a digestive enzyme. Unlike most digestive enzymes, bromelain is active both in the acid environment of the stomach and the alkaline environment of the small intestine. This may make it particularly effective as an oral digestive aid for those who do not digest food properly.
Bromelain may also increase the absorption of various drugs, particularly antibiotics such as amoxicillin and tetracycline. This could offer both risks and benefits.

While most large enzymes are broken down in the digestive tract, those found in bromelain appear to be absorbed whole to a certain extent. This finding makes it reasonable to suppose that bromelain can actually produce systemic (whole body) effects. Once in the blood, bromelain appears to reduce inflammation, "thin" the blood, and affect the immune system. These influences may be responsible for some of bromelain's therapeutic effects.

Bromelain appears to be essentially nontoxic, and it seldom causes side effects other than occasional mild gastrointestinal distress or allergic reactions.

Cherries

Raw, canned, cooked or in juice form, cherries have shown evidence of being able to reduce the pain and inflammation in joints for those suffering from lupus or rheumatoid arthritis, according to the University of Michigan Health System. The university reports that people who consumed about 8 oz. or 20 cherries daily for several weeks saw a significant reduction in pain and related joint symptoms. Any kind of cherries will do the trick; however, many people believe that sour cherries are more effective in lessening arthritis pain and inflammation. In addition to eating cherries, you can opt for drinking cherry juice. Again, tart cherry juice is often preferred over black cherry juice. Make sure the juice is unsweetened, or use cherry concentrate mixed with water, suggests "The People's Pharmacy Guide to Home and Herbal Remedies." Drinking two glasses daily during an acute attack may reduce symptoms, and then continue with one glass daily or alternate with 8 oz. of fresh cherries for variety.

Ginkgo Biloba

More commonly known as Ginkgo, is an herb that has been used for thousands of years in traditional Chinese medicine. This nutrient is often prepared by making an extract from the dried leaves. These extracts contain high concentrations of molecules called flavonoids and terpenoids, which are antioxidants and improve blood flow, respectively (McKenna, 2001).

A clinical study revealed that taking 120 mg of *Ginkgo biloba* extract three times per day for 10 weeks significantly reduced the number of Raynaud's phenomenon attacks, a set of symptoms that often affect people with lupus (Muir, 2002).

Green Tea Extract:

Researchers studied an animal model for type I diabetes and primary Sjogren's Syndrome, which damages the glands that produce tears and saliva.

They found significantly less salivary gland damage in a group treated with green tea extract, suggesting a reduction of the Sjogren's symptom commonly referred to as dry mouth. Dry mouth can also be caused by certain drugs, radiation and other diseases.

Since it is an autoimmune disease, Sjogren's Syndrome causes the body to attack itself and produce extra antibodies that mistakenly target the salivary and lacrimal glands. There is no cure or prevention for Sjogren's Syndrome.

Researchers studied the salivary glands of the water-consuming group and a green tea extract-consuming group to look for inflammation and the number of lymphocytes, a type of white blood cells that gather at sites of inflammation to fend off foreign cells.

The group treated with green tea had significantly fewer lymphocytes, Dr. Hsu says. Their blood also showed lower levels of autoantibodies, protein weapons produced when the immune system attacks itself, he says.

Researchers already know that one component of green tea – EGCG – helps suppress inflammation, according to Dr. Hsu. "So, we suspected that green tea would suppress the inflammatory response of this disease. Those treated with the green tea extract beginning at three weeks, showed significantly less damage to those glands over time."

Researchers also suspect that the EGCG in green tea can turn on the body's defense system against TNF-alpha – a group of proteins and molecules involved in systemic inflammation. TNF-alpha, which is produced by white blood cells, can reach out to target and kill cells.

"The salivary gland cells treated with EGCG had much fewer signs of cell death caused by TNF-alpha," Dr. Hsu says. "We don't yet know exactly how EGCG makes that happen. That will require further study. In some ways, this study gives us more questions than answers."

The University of Maryland Medical Center reports that compounds in green tea may lower the risk of certain forms of cancer, including malignancies of the lungs, breast, colon, bladder and prostate. However, according to the National Institutes of Health, there is not enough conclusive evidence to demonstrate green tea's ability to prevent cancer.

Dehydroepiandrosterone   (DHEA)
DHEA is a hormone naturally produced by the adrenal gland and is converted into sex hormones. In addition to being produced in the body, DHEA is also present in the Mexican yam, from which it is extracted for use as a nutritional supplement (Coates, 2010).

In a clinical trial, when individuals with lupus took 200 mg of DHEA daily for 24 weeks, the number of patients who experienced lupus flares was significantly reduced (Chang, 2002). In another study, the same investigators showed that taking 200 mg of DHEA daily for 24 weeks reduced blood levels of the cytokine IL-10, which enhances antibody production (Chang, 2004). This reduction in IL-10 may have contributed to the reduced incidence of lupus flares seen in the first study.

Another double-blind, randomized, controlled trial involving 41 women found that six months treatment with 20 – 30 mg DHEA daily improved mental and emotional well-being in lupus patients (Nordmark, 2005). Also, at a dose of 200 mg daily, DHEA improved bone mineral density in postmenopausal women with lupus (Hartkamp, 2004).

Vitamin E

Vitamin E is a fat-soluble vitamin that is stored in the liver and has powerful antioxidant activity, according to the Office of Dietary Supplements, or ODS. Antioxidants help protect cells from damage by free radicals that can lead to the onset of heart disease and cancer. The ODS reports that laboratory studies of vitamin E activity show that the antioxidant helps improve immune function. In a study published in the journal "Clinical Rheumatology" in March 2007, researchers found that about 150 to 300 mg per day of vitamin E, combined with other lupus medications, may interfere with key characteristics of the autoimmune disease.

Resveratrol

Resveratrol is a polyphenol antioxidant found in grapes, purple grape juice, red wine, peanuts, some berries and in supplement form. Resveratrol works in several ways to reduce inflammation. Researchers are beginning to understand the complex mechanisms of how resveratrol is effective for preventing   inflammation. One way resveratrol works is in suppressing prostaglandins. Prostaglandins are hormone-like substance made of fatty acids and are markers of inflammation. Sickness and infection within the body can cause a prostaglandin release, which is oftentimes what causes pain. Cardiovascular disease is characterized by the release of prostaglandins. Resveratrol acts to suppress prostaglandins in white blood cells and this may be how resveratrol is thought to be cardioprotective, according to a study in the 2006 journal "Comprehensive Reviews in Food Science and Food Safety."

Cytokines are protein molecules secreted by cells of the immune system. Cytokines contribute to inflammation in the body. Resveratrol prevents the inflammatory action of cytokines. An example of this was seen in a study published in the 2003 journal "Thorax," in which resveratrol prevented release of cytokines from cells in the lungs. These particular cells, known as alveolar macrophages, play a role in consuming inhaled particulate matter. The participants in the study were smokers and patients with chronic obstructive pulmonary disease.

Research from the Linus Pauling Institute (LPI) has reported that resveratrol is effective as neutralizing free radicals and other agents that promote cancer. Evidence-based studies show resveratrol inhibits the spread of cancer cells in several tissues such as breast, prostate, stomach and colon. In one trial, resveratrol administered orally was shown to halt the growth of esophageal, intestinal and breast cancer that are normally caused by carcinogens and other free radicals. Free radicals are harmful agents such as cigarette smoke and radiation that promote cancer cells.

Significant research from the Linus Pauling Institute, has seen a reduction in cardiovascular disease risk associated with moderate consumption of red wine. Red wine contains high levels of resveratrol and other flavonoids that researchers claim reduce the risk of heart disease and promote health. The LPI studies report that resveratrol is a powerful antioxidant that prevents inflammation that inhibits many diseases. Moderate alcohol consumption has been shown to reduce heart disease, but researchers believe that resveratrol provides additional benefits to heart health beyond those associated with alcohol. Several studies reported patients administered alcohol-free resveratrol noted significant improvements in several cardiovascular areas.

Reports from the Mayo Clinic suggest that resveratrol is the active proponent in red wine that is responsible for cardiovascular protection. It helps prevent damage by reducing inflammation in blood vessels, preventing clots, and reducing LDL, or "bad" cholesterol.

Most resveratrol supplements available in the U.S. contain extracts of the root of *Polygonum cuspidatum*, also known as Hu Zhang or kojo-kon . Red wine extracts and red grape extracts containing resveratrol and other polyphenols are also available in the U.S. as dietary supplements. Resveratrol supplements may contain anywhere from 10-50 mg of resveratrol, but the effective doses for chronic disease prevention in humans are not known, but a reasonable dose for autoimmunity is 300 mg daily. Please consult with your health care provider.

Turmeric

Turmeric, or curcumin, is a plant that is widely used as a spice in traditional curry dishes and is grown primarily in India and other parts of Asia. It is used in traditional Chinese medicine and Ayurvedic medicine. Turmeric is used to treat digestive and liver conditions, arthritis pain, irregular menstrual periods, heartburn, stomach ulcers and gallstones and is even used to prevent and treat certain types of cancer. It has natural anti-inflammatory qualities as well as blood-thinning properties.

Curcumin, a bioactive derivative of the spice turmeric, has been tested over the last several years for its antioxidant, anti-cancer, and anti-inflammatory clinical properties. Curcumin decreases the ability of lupus autoantibodies to bind their specific antigens an average of 52. The damaging inflammation of lupus-mediated injury is facilitated by the binding of autoantibodies to protein and nucleic acid antigens. Therefore, successful blocking of antigen/autoantibody binding suppresses inflammation before it even begins.

Experimental studies have revealed a considerable role for curcumin in modulating inflammatory cross-talk between cells of the immune system by suppressing cytokines such as IL-1beta, IL-6, IL-12 and TNFα (Bright, 2007). Moreover, a recent animal model of an autoimmune disease identified NFkβ suppression as a key mechanism behind curcumin's anti-inflammatory action.

A clinical trial tested the effects of curcumin in 24 patients with the lupus-associated kidney disease lupus nephritis. One group of patients took 500 mg of turmeric daily over a 3-month period, which is equivalent to a daily curcumin dose of 22.1 mg. Compared to the placebo control group, the turmeric group exhibited significant improvement in proteinuria (Khajehdehi ,2011).

Although some clinical studies have been conducted showing some signs and symptoms are reduced in some autoimmune diseases such as multiple sclerosis and rheumatoid arthritis, clinical studies have not yet been conducted to determine if curcumin has a similar effect with lupus (Bright, 2007). However, these results are promising and suggest potential beneficial effects of curcumin in people with lupus.

Numerous studies have looked into the connection between autoimmune diseases like lupus and various herbs and supplements like turmeric. A 2009 study published in "The International Journal of Biochemistry and Cell Biology," reports that curcumin, an antioxidant that is an active ingredient in turmeric, has shown to play a major role in the prevention and treatment of inflammatory autoimmune diseases such as lupus.

While turmeric is safe, you need to use caution if you take medications such as Coumadin to thin your blood. Because turmeric is a natural blood thinner, taking it together with Coumadin can increase your risks of bleeding and bruising. Let your physician know if you use turmeric in your regular diet, or supplements, as they may need to adjust your Coumadin prescription.

Synthetic Vs. Whole Food Supplements

Most retail brands are a waste of money. In fact, most over the counter brands are synthetic and contain impurities or additives that could actually make you worse. Now that vitamins have become a popular market, store shelves are filled with attractive bottles. Even 'health food' stores sometimes stock shelves with high-priced yet synthetic products. The cheapest brand is fine when it comes to products such as toilet paper or kleenex, but you are not ingesting those products.

A good assumption is that a vitamin or supplement will be synthetic unless otherwise noted. Whole foods supplements are more costly to manufacture so the makers of such vitamins will be sure to point it out so you will know why you're paying more money for their product. The majority of multi-vitamins you buy in stores are synthetic.

For example, look at this popular retail multivitamin label:

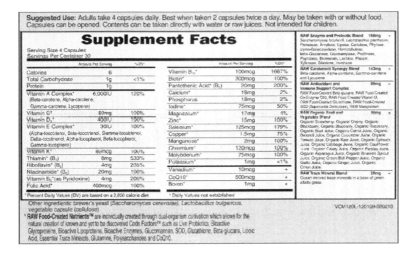

Yumm! Polyvinyl alcohol! Compare to a popular Whole Food Multivitamin label:

There is no such thing as a single molecule that makes up most vitamins. Whole food vitamins are actually groups of chemically-related compounds that cluster in the foods we eat. There are other, extremely important molecules associated with the major vitamins. These are the cofactors, trace minerals, co-enzymes, and anti-oxidants necessary for the whole food vitamin to work. If you choose a vitamin that is a whole food vitamin, you will get those extra factors along with the main clusters of vitamin molecules, increasing the ability of the vitamin to function. The whole food vitamins are easily absorbed, including the vitamin micronutrients that go with them.

In addition, they are completely in the form that the body needs them in. Our bodies know exactly how much of a specific vitamin is needed,and allows the rest to pass through the system. This is a process known as "selective absorption." Synthetic vitamins are missing these essential micronutrients. The body needs to find a way to match the synthetic vitamin with whatever micronutrients it can find. It also has to deal with these chemical vitamins much the same way that ity handles toxins and other unwanted chemicals, especially since they have no fuction without the support of other micronutriuents that are found in whole food supplements.

The metabolism of the unwanted synthetic vitamins can lead to vitamin overdoses and imbalances in body chemistry. Manufacturers cannot disassemble whole food complexes and turn them back into assembled complexes, because once a whole food vitamin complex has been disassembled into its component parts, it is considered "dead," and nonfunctional.

As you can imagine, taking part of a vitamin is not nearly as effective as taking the whole thing. For example, vitamin E loses 99% of its potency when separated from its natural whole food family. Vitamin E contains four different related tocopherols, plus xanthine, lipositols, and the mineral selenium. When you just take the tocopherols (which is the only part that is in synthetics), you throw out the real vitamin E. The tocopherols are nature's way of protecting the real vitamin E, much like skin on a fruit. In fact, its only a portion of real vitamin E and has only about 1% of the molecular activity of food vitamin E. If selenium isn't included, the vitamin E fragment is poorly absorbed and not utilized by the body. The body then becomes relatively diminished in its selenium content as it uses it up in an attempt to absorb the alpha-tocopherol.

Again, the problem can have a wide-ranging influence throughout the body. For example, selenium is necessary to convert T4 into T3 inside the liver. Without enough selenium, you can develop problems with your thyroid function because the active form of thyroid hormone, T3, is not being converted easily. I could go on and on, but then you would fall asleep! The main thing to remember is to look for "whole food supplement" on the label. Check out the Resource List at the end of the book for some examples.

Jenn's List of Essential Supplements for Autoimmunity

*Please consult with your health care provider before beginning this or any supplement program.

- Coenzyme Q10: 100mg daily
- Vitamin D3: 2,000-5,000 IU daily
- Vitamin C: 1,000-2,000 mg daily
- Dry Vitamin E: 300 IU daily
- Omega 3 Fatty Acids: 2,000-4,000 mg Daily
- Whole Food Vitamin Supplement (Rainbow Light Just Once, Garden of Life, are examples)

- Vitamin B Complex: 50mg daily
- Probiotic: at least 3 Billion cultures daily
- Green Tea Extract:500-1.500 mg of capsule form daily
- Tumeric (Curcumin) : 400 – 800 mg daily (as BCM-95-enhanced absorption curcumin)
- Ginkgo biloba; For Raynaud's: standardized extract: 120 – 360 mg daily
- DHEA—For Lupus: 50mg to start for 4 weeks; then 100 mg for 4 weeks, then 200 mg daily
- Zinc: 25-50mg Daily
- Resveratrol—150 mg twice daily

Thank you!

References:

Amital, H., et al., Serum concentrations of 25-OH vitamin D in patients with systemic lupus erythematosus (SLE) are inversely related to disease activity: is it time to routinely supplement patients with SLE with vitamin D? Annals of the rheumatic diseases, 2010.

Berdanier, C.D., J.T. Dwyer, and E.B. Feldman, Handbook of nutrition and food. 2nd ed 2008, Boca Raton: Taylor & Francis.

Borba, V.Z., et al., Vitamin D deficiency in patients with active systemic lupus erythematosus. Osteoporosis international : a journal established as result of cooperation between the European Foundation for Osteoporosis and the National Osteoporosis Foundation of the USA, 2009.

Bright, J.J., Curcumin and autoimmune disease. Advances in experimental medicine and biology, 2007.

Brown, A.C. Lupus erythematosus and nutrition: a review of the literature. Journal of Renal Nutrition, October 2000.

Cantorna, M.T. and B.D. Mahon, Mounting evidence for vitamin D as an environmental factor affecting autoimmune disease prevalence. Experimental biology and medicine, 2004.

Chang, D.M., et al., Dehydroepiandrosterone suppresses interleukin 10 synthesis in women with systemic lupus erythematosus. Annals of the rheumatic diseases, 2004.

Clark, W.F., et al., Fish oil in lupus nephritis: clinical findings and methodological implications. Kidney International, 1993.

Doria, A., et al., Risk factors for subclinical atherosclerosis in a prospective cohort of patients with systemic lupus erythematosus. Annals of the rheumatic diseases, 2003.

Hartkamp A et al. The effect of dehydroepiandrosterone on lumbar spine bone mineral density in patients with quiescent systemic lupus erythematosus. Arthritis Rheum. 2004.

Khajehdehi, P., et al., Oral Supplementation of Turmeric Decreases Proteinuria, Hematuria, and Systolic Blood Pressure in Patients Suffering from Relapsing or Refractory Lupus Nephritis: A Randomized and Placebo-controlled Study. Journal of renal nutrition : the official journal of the Council on Renal Nutrition of the National Kidney Foundation, 2011.

Lemire, J.M., Immunomodulatory role of 1,25-dihydroxyvitamin D3. Journal of cellular biochemistry, 1992.

National Center for Complementary and Alternative Medicine; The Use of Complementary and Alternative Medicine in the United States; December 2008.

McKenna, D.J., K. Jones, and K. Hughes, Efficacy, safety, and use of ginkgo biloba in clinical and preclinical applications. Alternative therapies in health and medicine, 2001.

Medical College of Georgia. Green Tea And EGCG May Help Prevent Autoimmune Diseases, 2007.

Muir, A.H., et al., The use of Ginkgo biloba in Raynaud's disease: a double-blind placebo-controlled trial. Vascular medicine, 2002.

Nordmark G et al. Effects of dehydroepiandrosterone supplement on health-related quality of life in glucocorticoid treated female patients with systemic lupus erythematosus. Autoimmunity. 2005

Sawalha AH et al. Dehydroepiandrosterone in systemic lupus erythematosus. Curr Rheumatol Rep. 2008.

Singh, U., S. Devaraj, and I. Jialal, Vitamin E, oxidative stress, and inflammation. Annual review of nutrition, 2005.

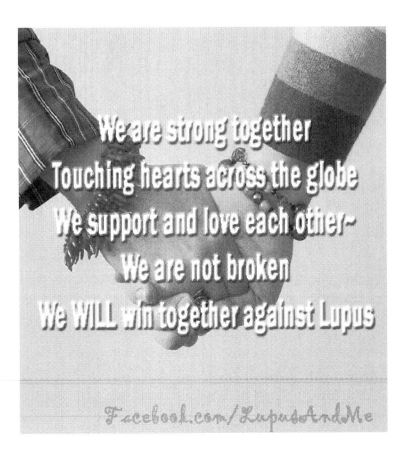

Resource List
Whole Food Vitamin Companies

The best whole food vitamins should meet certain standards for integrity and safety. A good vitamin supplement should be made according to pharmaceutical GMP, or Good Manufacturing Practice, which is the same compliance used by drug manufacturers enforced by the U.S. Food and Drug Administration. The best-rated vitamins should be labeled with the COA, or Certificate of Analysis, evidence of quality control testing. Also look for UPS on the label that ensures standards for strength, purity, disintegration and dissolution established by U.S. Pharmacopeia, according to MayoClinic. If your vitamin adheres to these standards, you know the supplement is a superior product, free from harmful contaminants and containing the actual ingredients listed.

Another reason to avoid chemically based vitamins is that they can actually increase rather than decrease the risks of chronic disease and side effects. A supplement containing alpha-tocopherol, beta-carotene, and selenium is known to chronically increase blood pressure. Vitamin C use as short as 6 weeks has been linked to excessive free radical activity. Vitamin E supplementation increases lung cancer and stroke risk, and overall mortality. Furthermore, the fat-soluble vitamins; A, D, E, and K, are stored in fat tissue and can cause symptoms of overdose if over-consumed for a long period. Examples include yellowing of the skin with beta-carotene, high triglyceride levels with vitamin A, and bleeding problems with vitamin E.

Whole food supplements are superior to vitamins in every way. Whole food supplements are comprised of concentrated portions of entire foods, not synthetic extracts. The advantage of these supplements is that you are getting a rich source of natural vitamins, but not so high that you are essentially overdosing. Also, whole food vitamins contain vitamins and

phytonutrients and many more cofactors and enzymes, which exponentially increase vitamin absorption in the body.
Some examples of proven whole foods vitamins (not all inclusive):

Garden of Life

Rainbow Light

New Chapter

The Vitamin Code

Juice Plus

Shaklee Vita Lea

Clean Eating

The Gracious Pantry

Clean Eating Magazine

The Paleo Solution: The Original Human Diet

Autoimmune Disorders

The Arthritis Foundation

Lupus Foundation of America

American Autoimmune Related Diseases Association

Hospital for Special Surgery Rheumatology

Dr Weil Autoimmune Articles

PubMed Health: Autoimmune Disorders

My Facebook page: www.facebook.com/LupusAndMe

Clean Eating Shopping List

PRODUCE

(choose in-season options)

Vegetables:

❑ Cucumber

❑ Romaine lettuce

❑ Mushrooms

❑ Green beans

❑ Asparagus

❑ Broccoli

❑ Squash

❑ Turnip

❑ Spinach

❑ Onions

❑ Garlic

❑ Celery

❑ Sweet Potatoes

❑ Potatoes

❑ Zucchini (baby squash)

❑ Tomato

Fruit

❑ Fresh berries (blueberries, blackberries,

raspberries, strawberries)

❑ Apples

❑ Bananas

❑ Pears

❑ Avocado

❑ Un-sweetened dried fruit (apricots,

cranberries, raisins, apples, prunes,

figs, dates)

BAKERY

❑ Whole-grain breads

❑ Brown rice wraps

❑ Whole-grain wraps (Ezekiel wraps)

MEAT, POULTRY,

SEAFOOD, & MEAT

ALTERNATIVES

❑ Chicken breast

❑ Pork tenderloin

❑ Salmon

❑ Tilapia, cod, or other white fish

❑ Firm and silken tofu

❑ Textured vegetable protein

❑ Beef tenderloin

❑ Bison

❑ Lean ground turkey

❑ Lean ground chicken

GROCERY LIST

DAIRY

❑ Eggs (omega-3 variety)

❑ Skim milk

❏ Fat-free soymilk, rice milk or almond milk

❏ Fat-free, sugar-free plain yogurt

❏ Olive oil-based margarine

❏ Kefir

NUTS, SEEDS, OILS,

AND SNACKS

❏ Unsalted almonds, cashews, walnuts

❏ Unsalted sunflower seeds

❏ All-natural nut & seed butters (almond,

cashew, peanut, tahini)

❏ Flaxseed

❏ Extra-virgin olive oil

❏ Safflower oil

❏ Pumpkin oil

❏ Pam (or non-stick spray)

❏ Other exotic oils

CEREALS

❏ Muesli

❏ Weetabix

❏ Kashi Go Lean

❏ Shredded Wheat

❏ All-Bran

❏ Steel-cut oats

❏ Cream of Wheat

DRY GOODS

❏ Brown rice

❏ Wheat germ

❏ Oats

❏ Oat bran

❏ Quinoa

❏ Bulgur

❏ Millet

❏ Baking soda

❏ Whole-wheat flour

- ❏ Baking powder
- ❏ Vanilla, best quality
- ❏ Sea salt
- ❏ Sugar substitute (Agave nectar, Sucanat,
  Rapadura, stevia)
- ❏ Other whole-grain flours (quinoa,
  amaranth, spelt)
- ❏ Spices (cumin, nutmeg, cinnamon)

CANNED GOODS

- ❏ Chickpeas
- ❏ Beans (navy, white, kidney, etc.)
- ❏ Lentils
- ❏ Tomatoes (crushed or whole)
- ❏ Water-packed tuna
- ❏ Water-packed salmon
- ❏ Low-fat, sugar-free, low-sodium soups

- ❏ Low-sodium corn and peas
- ❏ Tomato paste
- ❏ Low-sodium chicken or vegetable stock

CONDIMENTS

- ❏ Mustard
- ❏ Salsa
- ❏ All-natural, sugar-free tomato sauce
- ❏ Unsweetened, organic applesauce
- ❏ Honey

BEVERAGES

- ❏ Green tea
- ❏ Maca tea
- ❏ Tulsi tea
- ❏ Coffee
- ❏ Bottled water

MISCELLANEOUS

- ❏ Balsamic vinegar

❏ Rice vinegar   ❏ _____

❏ Lemon juice   ❏ _____

❏ Lime juice   ❏ _____

❏ Apple cider vinegar   ❏

_____

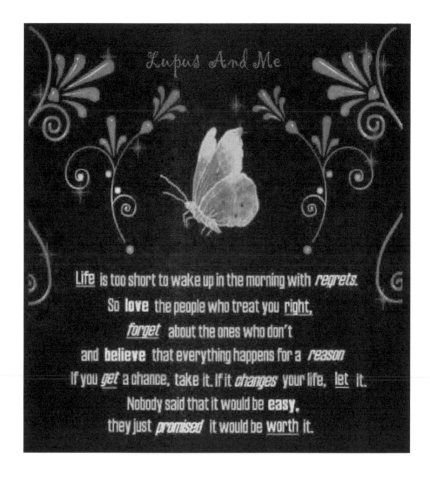

Notes

Notes

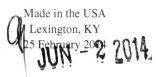

Made in the USA
Lexington, KY
25 February 2014